Backed by extensive research, Hanley and de Irala explore "risk reduction" and "risk avoidance" approaches to the prevention of AIDS in Africa. They succinctly identify the philosophies and agendas underpinning these approaches, question Western assumptions, and challenge the AIDS Establishment to give due acknowledgment to the effectiveness of abstinence and fidelity in AIDS prevention. The authors understand that faithful human love is the most effective promoter of health and wholeness.

SISTER MIRIAM DUGGAN, F.M.S.A., F.R.C.O.G.
Founder, Miriam Duggan Home
Kampala, Uganda

Deep respect for life and responsible sexuality are essential for integral human development. When Pope Benedict XVI calls for the humanization of sexuality, he has in mind the kind of arguments that Hanley and de Irala present in this book with such clarity, coherence, and conviction.

REV. MICHAEL CZERNY, S.J.
Founder and Director
African Jesuit AIDS Network
Nairobi, Kenya

The ruthless promotion of condoms by Western governments and international organizations is responsible for millions of deaths in Africa from AIDS-related diseases. Those in the Western world who want to overcome the tremendous crisis of HIV/AIDS that is devastating sub-Saharan Africa should ponder and take to heart the powerful message of Hanley and de Irala.

BISHOP HUGH SLATTERY, M.S.C.
Diocese of Tzaneen
South Africa

Affirming Love,
Avoiding AIDS

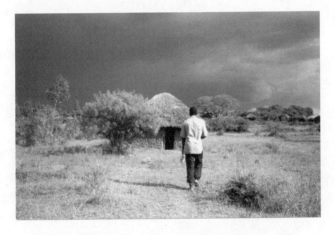

Phillip, a father of three and volunteer community health worker, brings bread, comfort, and company to a man with AIDS in his home near Lake Victoria in western Kenya, where close to a third of the population is HIV positive.

Affirming Love, Avoiding AIDS

What Africa Can Teach the West

MATTHEW HANLEY

JOKIN DE IRALA

WITH A FOREWORD BY EDWARD C. GREEN

THE NATIONAL CATHOLIC BIOETHICS CENTER

Philadelphia

Cover design by Nicholas Furton
Photograph on page iv by Matthew Hanley
ISBN 978-0-935372-56-4

An earlier version of this book was published in Spanish as *Propontelo, proponselo: evitar el SIDA* by Ediciones Internacionales Universitarias, 2006.

Unless otherwise noted, quotations from Church documents are from the Vatican English translation, published online at www .vatican.va.

Library of Congress Cataloging-in-Publication Data

Hanley, Matthew.

Affirming love, avoiding AIDS : what Africa can teach the West / Matthew Hanley, Jokin De Irala ; with a foreword by Edward C. Green.

p. ; cm.

An earlier version of this book was published in Spanish as Propontelo, proponselo: evitar el SIDA, by Ediciones Internacionales Universitarias, 2006.A

Includes bibliographical references and index.

ISBN 978-0-935372-56-4

1. AIDS (Disease)--Africa. 2. AIDS (Disease)--Religious aspects--Catholic Church. I. Irala, Jokin de. II. Hanley, Matthew. Propontelo, proponselo : evitar el SIDA. III. National Catholic Bioethics Center. IV. Title.

[DNLM: 1. Acquired Immunodeficiency Syndrome--prevention & control. 2. Christianity. 3. Sexual Behavior. WC 503.6 H241a 2010]

RA643.86.A25H36 2010

362.196'97920096--dc22

2010002609

*This book is dedicated to all who suffer anguish
from the HIV/AIDS epidemic
and to those who care for them and remain for them
a compassionate human presence.*

CONTENTS

❧·❧

FOREWORD

Future historians of the AIDS era will puzzle over and debate the reasons why spending ten billion dollars annually by 2007 seemed to have so little effect on global HIV infection rates. Specifically, when dealing with a disease that can be so easily prevented, why did efforts not go toward changing the behaviors that drive HIV epidemics, namely, having many sexual partners (especially those that are concurrent), the injection of mood-altering drugs, prostitution, and intercourse among homosexual men? Future historians will rightly conclude that special-interest groups presided over the rise of a vast multi-billion-dollar enterprise and focused it almost exclusively on the distribution of medical devices and drugs.

Serious efforts to change high-risk behaviors have been conspicuously missing in the effort to control AIDS. Put another way, there has been little or no primary prevention in HIV/AIDS, even though public and private sectors have poured more money and resources into this single disease than into any other in history. Efforts to include primary prevention are often rejected, surprisingly, in the name of achieving a so-called comprehensive approach to reducing the spread of HIV. Moreover, the heavy emphasis on "risk reduction," greatly facilitated by invoking the name of human rights, has also been regularly cast as the "scientific" course of action, thus requiring a monopoly of resource allocation. That drum has been beaten with great urgency, as though the inclusion of primary prevention messages would cause the comprehensive preventive paradigm to crumble and lead to an even greater pandemic.

How did the world's great experts in HIV/AIDS and allied fields get so far off course? How did they manage to convince themselves, the rest of the scientific and international development establishments, liberal churches, the mass media, and indeed most of the world that they were doing the right thing?

Let me mention one basic reason.[1] The global response to AIDS was developed by Americans (with some European input) for the type of "concentrated" HIV epidemics found in America and Europe. We then attempted to apply Euro-American solutions to problems in Africa, Asia, the Caribbean, and indeed the rest of the world. The great majority of HIV epidemics are concentrated among high-risk groups, usually among the universal risk groups of homosexual men, injecting drug users, and prostitutes. Yet a majority of the world's HIV infections are found in Africa among general populations, that is, not in these high-risk groups. In 2007, Africa accounted for 67 percent of all people living with AIDS and 75 percent of all AIDS deaths.

The Euro-American approach has its own flaws. First of all, prevention tools, aimed at reducing risk or harm among homosexual men and injecting drug users, have not been very successful even in concentrated epidemics. For example, HIV incidence appears to be rising again in the United States, and it has certainly risen in recent years among homosexual men, the risk group that contributes the highest proportion of HIV infections to the U.S. epidemic. But however effective risk reduction has been in concentrated epidemics, it should have occurred to AIDS experts that we need different approaches when most HIV infections are found in general populations. An approach that may be effective for a drug addict or a prostitute—which is based on the ultimately self-defeating premise that the risk behavior cannot (or even should not) be changed—will probably not be the best approach for married couples or most teenagers. After all, the majority of unmarried teenagers in less-developed countries are not sexually active, to go by our best behavioral surveys.[2]

There are several other reasons why global AIDS prevention got started on the wrong track, but let us look at what has worked. We probably now know the answer to this for at least the "hyper-epidemics" of Africa. These have been reduced by behavior change of a more fundamental sort than adoption of condoms or other technologies, or testing. In every African country where HIV infections have declined, this decline has been associated with a decrease in the proportion of men and women reporting more than one sex partner over the course of a year—which is exactly what fidelity programs promote.[3] The same association with HIV decline cannot be said for condom use, coverage of HIV testing, treatment for curable sexually transmitted infections, provision of antiretroviral drugs, or any other intervention or behavior.

The other behavior that has often been associated with a decline in HIV prevalence is a decrease in premarital sex among young people, but the evidence for this is not as strong as the evidence for partner reduction, nor does abstinence or delay of sexual debut involve as great a proportion of those between the ages of fifteen and forty-nine (where we track HIV infections and behavioral trends) who are sexually active.

It is quite possible that condom use also contributes to declines in HIV infection rates, but it is hard to know for certain. We might learn that condom use "in last high-risk encounter" or with last "nonregular partner" rose from, say, 40 to 60 percent, but the great majority of that condom use is irregular, and a growing body of research findings show that irregular condom use does not help overall.[4] In fact, it might actually contribute to higher levels of infection because of the phenomenon of risk compensation, whereby people take greater sexual risks because they feel safer than they really ought to because they are using condoms at least some of the time.[5] This is a complex and controversial issue that has generally been underappreciated, but Hanley and de Irala fairly and concisely pull together the evidence and profitably discuss its implications.

In fact, the only type of condom use that is really associated with risk reduction is *consistent* condom use. One of my criticisms of the AIDS Establishment in 2003 was that the major surveys we were relying on to inform and guide our AIDS prevention programs, such as the Demographic and Health Survey funded by the U.S. government, did not ask about consistent condom use, even though the word condom was used in questions twenty-nine times.[6] Perhaps because of criticism like my own, along with the landmark study of condom effectiveness by Norman Hearst and Sanny Chen,[7] the Demographic and Health Survey began asking a question about consistent condom use in 2005. Yet to date, the findings have not been published, analyzed, or discussed.

My guess is that when the data on consistent condom use are finally made available, levels of consistent use will prove to be so low as to make the billions of dollars poured into condom promotion look ill spent as well as ill monitored. And we will see that consistent condom use is especially rare in general populations, where most infections in Africa are found, in spite of all the efforts that have gone into promoting condoms to married couples, teenagers, and others in the general population. Even among discordant couples (where one partner is HIV positive and one is uninfected) who know their HIV status and have access to condoms, consistent condom use is rare.[8]

Under optimal conditions, condoms reduce risk of HIV infection by about 85 percent, but of course conditions are not usually optimal.

Hanley and de Irala also point out other facts that are not well known or publicized by the popular media. For example, even in countries like Thailand and Cambodia, where HIV infections are concentrated among prostitutes and their clients, declines in HIV infection rates, typically depicted as resulting exclusively from condom use, have also been attributed to declines in the proportion of men having contact with sex workers and to declines in the proportion of men having more than a single sex partner.

Those Catholics who are agonizing over a perceived disconnect between Church teaching on condom use and effective AIDS prevention will benefit from reading Hanley and de Irala's book. Firmly planted on solid epidemiological ground, their work stands in sharp relief to many others in the faith-based community who have curiously adopted a politically correct and unsubstantiated viewpoint that is virtually indistinguishable from what one might expect to find at thoroughly secularized institutions. If anything, we should have learned from the evidence alone that to make a constructive contribution to global AIDS control, one does not need to jettison core beliefs related to sexual restraint or imply (as some Church-affiliated entities have done) that the epidemic stems primarily from outdated moral teachings which principally serve to foster stigma and discrimination.

Yet the Church, and in fact all religious groups and leaders, can be as misled by the experts as everyone else. It is not surprising that compassionate and well-meaning people of faith sometimes end up supporting ineffective types of AIDS prevention when they are assured by scientists and the mass media that condoms are the best weapon we have in the war against AIDS, that abstinence and fidelity or monogamy are not feasible and may even be "impossible" and, even more remarkably, that marriage is in fact a dangerous enterprise for women in the developing world. For example, Nicholas Kristof wrote in the *New York Times* that "just about the deadliest thing a woman in South Africa can do is get married."[9] In 2009, the chairman of the Uganda AIDS Commission testified before UNAIDS that marriage has somehow emerged as a major risk factor for AIDS.[10] I am afraid he has been led astray by foreign donors who want to keep the focus on condoms. The truth is that married people in Africa are always found to have lower HIV infection rates than people who are single, divorced, or widowed, when comparing the same age groups (except for the comparison between married teenage females and unmarried teens, most of whom are abstaining). Allison Herling and I discussed this issue in some detail in an article published by *First Things*, in which we identify "the central fact that has emerged from all the recent studies of the HIV epidemic: What the churches are called to do by their theology turns out to be what works best in AIDS prevention."[11] We are referring of course to the promotion of marital fidelity and premarital abstinence.

Hanley and de Irala cover the evidence that has been debated bitterly in recent years, and they show how fidelity and abstinence are in fact not faith-based motivational programs but evidence-based AIDS prevention. They cover in some detail the evidence for what brought down HIV infection rates in Uganda so dramatically. In my own research I have found that the Catholic Church has played a significant role not only in caring for the sick and dying, but also in AIDS prevention. An Irish medical missionary, Sister Dr. Miriam Duggan, F.M.S.A., was a key figure in the development and shaping of Uganda's distinctive prevention program that put primary emphasis on marital fidelity and delay of sexual debut.

One of the notable Catholic AIDS prevention programs is Youth Alive, which has had to struggle financially because most of the major donors have refused to fund an AIDS program that does not promote and distribute condoms. As I reported in a study I conducted for the U.S. Agency for International Development,

> Youth Alive emphasizes "the spiritual approach to life" as well as to AIDS. "We are dealing with such great problems as stigma, shame, depression and loss of loved ones that come with this disease. You cannot take care of this with a condom. You need spiritual and social support." The program director explained, "When I say A, B, C, to us as a church, the C is for character formation for the youth, and not condom."

> One informant put it this way. "If you elevate the condom to the highest good, then you are saying or implying that people are only animals who cannot

reason and who cannot control their biological urges." "We teach that people are more than that, that they are intelligent, worthy, valuable, loved by God." Another comment was "We have a belief that each and every individual has the capacity to change."[12]

It is seldom mentioned, but the major HIV/AIDS organizations do not really agree with this last statement. Every reason is given to argue that poor people in particular do not have the freedom, the "agency," the power, or the opportunity to fundamentally change sexual behavior—except for adopting certain technologies that we on the donor side can provide. This attitude quite naturally serves selfish financial interests, even as it also reflects often passionate ideological commitments to the sexual freedom and license enshrined by the Western sexual revolution.

But Hanley and de Irala convincingly point out that this position is fundamentally one born of despair, and one which inevitably shortchanges the very people our prevention programs strive to protect. In fact, after discussing the scientific questions on their own empirical terms, Hanley and de Irala present and contrast the Christian perspective on these matters with the prevailing secular perspective, discussing in some detail the competing visions of the person and of human sexuality, and the role of holding out hope for a better future. Here they make their most creative contribution to the global AIDS debates by providing a glimpse of what, beneath all the rhetoric, ultimately drives much of AIDS prevention policy, and contrasting it with a positive, rational articulation of the unpopular Catholic teachings that are frequently misunderstood or misrepresented.

If I may be permitted to end on a personal note, I went through a very difficult period after coming to Harvard in 2001 and speaking out from that bully pulpit about how and why our AIDS prevention approach was not working well. Especially during the years 2002 to 2005, I was making many presentations to audiences at the U.S. Agency for International Development, at reproductive health and family planning associations and conventions, in the House of Representatives and the U.S. Senate, and elsewhere. Matt Hanley would often be in the audience, at times possibly the only person present who really supported my viewpoint. He would usually come up to me after I had received a chilly reception and say a few words of encouragement. This was important for me, because I had been raised to think that if I thought one way about some issue and everyone else thought the opposite way, both common sense and a modicum of humility would suggest that it was I who was wrong. Matt's presence reminded me that sometimes the majority of experts can be wrong.

EDWARD C. GREEN

Edward Green is the director of the AIDS Prevention Research Project at the Harvard Center for Population and Development Studies in Cambridge, Massachusetts.

Notes

1. I address this question in my forthcoming book, *AIDS and Ideology* (Sausilito, CA: PoliPoint Press, 2010).

2. "Abstinence of Never-Married Young Men and Women," HIV/AIDS Survey Indicators Database, November 16, 2009, http://www.measuredhs.com/hivdata/data/, available from the author.

3. Edward C. Green and Allison Herling, *The ABC Approach to Preventing the Sexual Transmission of HIV: Common Questions and Answers* (Morgantown, PA: Masthof Press, 2006).

4. Saifuddin Ahmed et al. "HIV Incidence and Sexually Transmitted Disease Prevalence Associated with Condom Use: A Population Study in Rakai, Uganda," *AIDS* 15.16 (November 9, 2001): 2171–2179; and James D. Shelton, "Ten Myths and One Truth about Generalised HIV Epidemics," *Lancet* 370.9602 (December 1, 2007): 1809–1811.

5. Phoebe Kajubi et al., "Increasing Condom Use without Reducing HIV Risk: Results of a Controlled Community Trial in Uganda," *Journal of Acquired Immune Deficiency Syndromes* 40.1 (September 1, 2005): 77–82; and Michael M. Cassell et al., "Risk Compensation: The Achilles' Heel of Innovations in HIV Prevention?" *British Medical Journal* 332.7541 (2006): 605–607.

6. Edward C. Green, *Rethinking AIDS Prevention: Learning from Successes in Developing Countries* (Santa Barbara: CA, Praeger, 2003).

7. Norman Hearst and Sanny Chen, "Condom Promotion for AIDS Prevention in the Developing World: Is It Working?" *Studies in Family Planning* 35.1 (March 2004): 39–47.

8. Ibid.

9. Nicholas D. Kristof, "When Marriage Kills," *New York Times*, March 30, 2005, http://www.nytimes.com/2005/03/30/opinion/30kristof.html.

10. Charles Wendo, "Uganda: New HIV Cases Alarm Doctors," *New Vision*, January 8, 2009, http://allafrica.com/stories/2009 01090004.html.

11. Edward C. Green and Allison Herling Ruark, "AIDS and the Churches: Getting the Story Straight," *First Things* 182 (April 2008): 22–26.

12. Edward C. Green, *Case Studies of ABC: Models for the Implementation of Abstinence and 'Faithfulness' Behavior Change Programs* (Cambridge, MA: USAID and Harvard School of Public Health, 2003), especially p. 25. This unpublished study is available at http://www.ccih.org/resources/ABCplus/research/abc/case-studies-of-ABC.pdf.

I

The ABC Approach

The initial attempts to deal with the HIV/AIDS epidemic in Africa have been, many experts now think, a "public health failure."[1] It is thus vital that public health authorities take a fresh look at the principal strategies and policies that have long been favored for containing the epidemic. This examination may help them reorient these strategies to better correspond to the behavioral dynamics of HIV transmission.

The failure to contain HIV is even more striking because almost all the Western institutional actors with power to shape policy, direct funding, and implement programs have shared the firm conviction that technically oriented risk reduction strategies (primarily, but not solely, the promotion of condom use) must be the unequivocal HIV prevention priority. We will at times refer to these influential actors as the AIDS Establishment. By this we mean global authorities like the World Health Organization and UNAIDS (the Joint United Nations Program on HIV/AIDS) as well as powerful and diffuse Western governmental donor agencies like USAID (the U.S. Agency for International Development) and its European counterparts. These institutions create policy guidelines and fund initiatives to carry out their strategic priorities. Nongovernmental organizations, which are often dependent on governmental funding for their survival and frequently share the donor's worldview, collaborate by carrying out donor agency priorities, sometimes called "best practices" even if their track record has been flimsy. Many NGOs specialize in "family planning" services, particularly the distribution of contraceptives.

Academics from prestigious universities and a range of activists' interest groups also form an important part of the AIDS Establishment. Leading medical and scientific journals often show a strong editorial preference for reports based on the technically oriented approach to HIV prevention favored by the AIDS Establishment.

Some individuals within these institutions have managed to create space outside the dominant HIV prevention paradigm for discouraging the actual behaviors driving HIV transmission. They have made enormous contributions. Nonetheless, the AIDS Establishment's overwhelming HIV prevention emphasis has remained technical as opposed to behavioral.

The most recognizable example of a policy shift which made room for behavioral strategies occurred when USAID adopted the ABC approach to HIV prevention in recognition of the success of Uganda's response to the AIDS epidemic.[2] The A of ABC stands for *abstinence* and refers to education and support for people to postpone sexual initiation and to avoid sporadic sexual relations. The B stands for *be faithful* and represents the recommendation to have mutually monogamous sexual relations with an uninfected person. The C stands for *condom use*, based on the knowledge that condoms may reduce the risk of infection but will not eliminate the risk altogether.

We now know that fundamental changes in sexual behavior, particularly declines in multiple sexual partnerships, are what have led to every instance of falling HIV rates in Africa. Indeed, changes in primary sexual behavior are always found when HIV/AIDS prevalence declines.[3] Based on considerable evidence indicating the indispensable role that behavior plays in practice, particularly in Africa, we are convinced that more explicit emphasis on risk avoidance is warranted. By *risk avoidance* we mean public health interventions that stress abstinence (A) and fidelity (B), as opposed to risk reduction interventions that stress condom use (C) and related technical measures.

From an epidemiological point of view, this shift would help everywhere, although it would have the greatest impact, and is thus most urgently needed, in regions with generalized epidemics. From a philosophical point of view, it would offer a far superior service to the human person, who is the subject of and principal agent of his or her own development, and to whom all public health measures should be directed. From the public health point of view, it would represent a commonsense return to the discipline's bedrock disease control principle: primary prevention.

We will examine the epidemiological record, high-lighting countries that have successfully reversed their HIV epidemics, and describe the behaviors to which that reversal is most attributable. These successes will be contrasted with the record of the three main pillars of HIV prevention strategy favored by the AIDS Establishment, each of which is aimed at risk reduction: condom use, voluntary counseling and testing, and the treatment of other sexually transmitted infections. Given the burden and severity of the epidemic in Africa, our attention will be focused there.

We acknowledge that we are sketching in broad strokes, that experience varies, and that fair-minded observers can interpret the data differently. Determining the efficacy and the epidemiological impact of interventions can sometimes be complex. But the data, derived from the evidence base, are nonetheless formidable and deserve to be evaluated on their own terms. Instances of clear success in reducing HIV prevalence have been relatively few, yet they offer our greatest cause for hope and remind us of the inherent human capacity to change behavior.

While the debate over HIV prevention has often been cast in "scientific" terms, it is better understood as a debate between two moral and philosophical approaches to human sexuality. On the one hand there is the broad Judeo-Christian tradition, which celebrates the gift of sexuality within the institution of marriage. This tradition recognizes moral boundaries as instruments of human fulfillment and well-being, not oppression. In practice it requires a measure of sacrifice, or self-restraint; it also recognizes that sexual expression can be destructive when limits are not respected. In short, it recognizes natural law.

Modern Western culture, on the other hand, fiercely resists this moral vision (with its inherent constraints), and attempts to replace it with other ideological currents and substitute creeds. Culture, like nature, abhors a vacuum. Modern Western culture exalts absolute freedom, understood as the abolition of limits in the autonomous pursuit of pleasure. If nature were simply allowed to run its course, this vision would be self-defeating, and so it requires an enabling ally in the form of "safety." This explains the determined quest for technical means of preempting undesirable consequences of sexual activity.

The individual's pursuit of pleasure is protected by the modern West's ultimate cultural code of silence: dogmatic nonjudgmentalism. To claim that there is indeed an objective moral order or "code of conduct," or even to argue that that code is designed for the good of the human person, is not only discomfiting but unpardonable: it gives offense. In the second half of this book we offer some reflections on HIV risk avoidance from a Christian perspective, in contrast to secular philosophical perspectives.

In this book we first present the relevant scientific data and only then examine the Christian and other philosophical approaches to HIV prevention. The exception comes in our treatment of behavioral disinhibition, or "risk compensation," since both religious leaders and scientists have voiced concern that promoting condoms may actually foster a false sense of security and lead to increased risk-taking behavior and vulnerability. It seems appropriate in this case to present the relevant scientific data and religious commentary side by side. We very much welcome a dialogue in which questions of science are engaged on their own terms, and questions about the ethical and moral dimensions of sexual behavior are likewise engaged on their own terms.

Approximately 27 percent of people with AIDS are being cared for by the Catholic Church throughout the world. No other single entity provides more for those suffering from or affected by AIDS. In addition to the Church's extensive experience in caring for and supporting the sick, it also has its own internally consistent and legitimate views on HIV prevention and human sexuality. What the Church holds to be true in these matters is not exclusively Catholic; rather, it is a position shared by many people, those of other faiths and those outside faith communities, and it is open to all by the use of ordinary human reason.

Any imprecision in our presentation of the Christian perspective is our own and will gladly be acknowledged and corrected subject to the proper teaching authorities.

Notes

1. M.A. Martinez-Gonzalez and Jokin de Irala, "Preventive Medicine and the Catastrophic Failures of Public Health: We Fail Because We Are Late" [in Spanish], *Medicina Clínica* 124.17 (May 7, 2005): 656–660.

2. Janice A. Hogle, ed., *What Happened in Uganda? Declining HIV Prevalence, Behavior Change and the National Response*

(Washington, D.C.: U.S. Agency for International Development, September 2002), http://www.usaid.gov/pop_health/aids/Countries/africa/uganda_report.pdf.

3. T. Stammers, "As Easy as ABC? Primary Prevention of Sexually Transmitted Infections," *Postgraduate Medicine Journal* 81.955 (May 2005): 273–275.

II

A Relentless Crisis

Acquired immune deficiency syndrome, or AIDS, is caused by the retrovirus HIV, or human immunodeficiency virus. The virus damages the immune systems of infected persons and leaves them susceptible to opportunistic infections and tumors. Treatment with antiretroviral drugs can slow the progress of the disease, but cannot cure it.

HIV is transmitted primarily by sexual contact or by sharing needles or syringes with an infected person. It is transmitted to a lesser extent through transfusions of infected blood or blood products, although this is now rare in countries where blood and blood derivatives are controlled. Babies born to infected mothers can become infected before or during birth, and by breastfeeding.

Because the virus does not survive well in the environment, its transmission in the home or workplace is extremely rare when universal precautions are implemented: usage of gloves, protection of wounds, avoidance of sharing razors or toothbrushes, and appropriate use and disposal of needles and syringes. There is no documented evidence of transmission by exposure to the saliva, tears, or sweat of an infected person, despite the presence of the virus in these fluids. (Nevertheless, kissing with the mouth open should be avoided to prevent contact with blood and saliva through tiny sores.[1]) Insects such as mosquitoes have not been known to transmit the disease.

There is not really one illness or one clinical manifestation of an illness arising from HIV infection. Rather, there is a gradual progression from initial HIV infection, through subsequent deterioration of the immune system, to the eventual development of AIDS. Initial HIV infection may or may not be accompanied by a short period of acute symptoms similar to those of infectious mononucleosis, which include fever, muscle aches, sore throat, and lymph node inflammation. Once persons are infected with HIV, they can never completely rid themselves of the virus, and there is currently no cure.

Infected persons are said to have become HIV positive, which is not necessarily equivalent to having AIDS. HIV-positive persons typically live with HIV for several years, often with few symptoms, before their immunity falls so low that they develop AIDS. Today many more people have HIV than have AIDS; everyone with AIDS is HIV positive. However, it is important to note that the virus may be transmitted from an HIV-positive person to another person at any time, even if the HIV-positive person is asymptomatic or does not yet have full-blown AIDS.

The initial phase of HIV infection has important implications for HIV prevention. Soon after the virus enters the body, it begins to replicate itself rapidly; in the process the virus attacks and suppresses immune cells known as CD4 cells. This spike in the HIV viral load and the destruction of immune (CD4) cells account for the morbidity a person experiences during that window of time, typically a few months immediately following HIV infection. The heightened viral load also makes the person more infectious to others during that period.

After the initial phase of HIV infection, the body responds by producing enough CD4 cells to replace those destroyed by the HIV virus. This has a stabilizing effect and ushers in the intermediate phase of HIV infection. This phase can last anywhere from several months to several years and is often characterized by a lack of symptoms.

Gradually, however, the rate of HIV viral replication and CD4 destruction exceeds that of CD4 production, and disease progression intensifies. An HIV-positive person develops a clinical AIDS diagnosis when their immunity, as measured by the quantity of CD4 cells, drops below a certain level. They may also be presumed to have AIDS if they develop an AIDS-defining illness, irrespective of official CD4 count or determination of HIV status.

There are several broad categories of AIDS-defining illnesses. One such category is called "opportunistic infections," caused when pathogens such as bacteria and viruses that would normally be repelled by a fully functioning immune system are able to take hold because of the weakened immunity of the HIV-positive person. Opportunistic infections associated with HIV infection include tuberculosis, pneumonia, and candidiasis. It is not uncommon, particularly in the developing world, for people to discover their HIV status only at this point. Those with AIDS often experience weight loss, fever, and diarrhea as well. AIDS in an advanced stage is often characterized by the appearance of tumors like Kaposi's sarcoma, serious infections in any organ of the body, AIDS-related wasting, or a combination of these.

The lag time between an initial HIV infection and the subsequent development of AIDS has at times challenged health authorities and the media alike to find terminology that reflects the continuum of disease progression or the extent of the problem in a given population. At one time AIDS authorities began to counsel the use of the term HIV/AIDS, as opposed to simply AIDS, to highlight the fact that there are many people living with HIV who have not yet developed AIDS. After all, many HIV-positive people are active and appear perfectly healthy. In fact, most HIV-positive people in countries with severe epidemics do not even know they have it. Actual AIDS cases represent the tip of the iceberg, while the cases of those with HIV or at risk of becoming HIV positive were the mountain of ice beneath the surface. Using the two acronyms HIV/AIDS side by side was meant to raise awareness of that reality; it was not meant to blur the distinctions between the virus and the syndrome it causes. In recent years, as treatment has become more widely available and people live with HIV for longer periods of time, AIDS authorities have chosen to separate the terms somewhat, speaking of "HIV and AIDS" in order to draw out further the distinctions in the continuum of disease progression.

Certainly there are times when the use of "HIV" alone or "AIDS" alone is most accurate, and other times when it is preferable to refer to them together ("HIV and AIDS"). It is thus customary now to speak of preventing the transmission of HIV (though this too is a bit of an oversimplification, since preventing HIV transmission also averts AIDS cases) and of treating people with HIV and AIDS (by treating an HIV-positive person, progression to AIDS may be delayed). Nonetheless, the term "AIDS prevention" has long been accepted and is still commonly used and understood.

Describing the epidemic as a whole also poses similar challenges; for the better part of a decade it was referred to as the HIV/AIDS epidemic. Epidemiological studies often try to estimate the number of people living with HIV, the number newly infected with HIV over a given period of time (incidence), and the percentage of a given population living with HIV (prevalence), not all of whom have AIDS at the time of the study.

Just as there is no one illness, the larger picture is not so much a monolithic "global pandemic" as a constellation of epidemics with distinct transmission patterns. In some parts of the world—notably Eastern Europe and parts of

Asia—the virus is transmitted primarily through intravenous drug use; in other epidemics, primarily through homosexual contact; in others, through commercial "sex work."

Globally, approximately half of all new infections occur in southern Africa, a region with less than 3 percent of the world's population.[2] There, multiple sexual partnerships—specifically, concurrent multiple partnerships—drive the epidemic. These behavioral patterns are inherently dangerous, because "as soon as one person in a network of concurrent relationships contracts HIV, everyone else in the network is placed at risk."[3]

The lack of male circumcision helps account for the severity of some epidemics in southern and eastern Africa. Three randomized controlled trials, published in 2006 and early 2007, concluded that male circumcision confers a partial but significant degree of protection for men against HIV transmission.[4] Although this is an important variable, we will not deal directly with this issue, since we are focusing on the behavioral dimensions of HIV transmission and their implications for prevention.

A Deadly Threat

Since it was first identified in 1981, AIDS has been responsible for more than twenty-five million deaths; HIV has infected approximately 65 million human beings.[5] It is the world's fourth leading cause of lost years of life and avoidable deaths. According to the December 2007 UNAIDS report, by the end of 2007 approximately

33.2 million people in the world were living with HIV/AIDS. In 2007, about 6,800 people became infected every day (about 2.5 million in total) and approximately 6,000 people a day died. Approximately 40 percent of the new infections occurred in young people between fifteen and twenty-four years of age.[6]

The devastating effect of this epidemic can be seen in the decline in life expectancy in Africa. A person born in Zambia or Malawi in 2004 can expect to live 37.4 or 39.6 years, respectively,[7] compared with the average of 70 to 85 years in the West. The thirty-year decrease in life expectancy in Botswana between 1990 and 2002, due mainly to AIDS, is unprecedented in the history of the human race.[8]

Thirty-four percent of pregnant women in Botswana and 44 percent in Swaziland are infected with HIV. At these rates, even the most efficient and well-planned diagnostic and treatment services may be unable to handle the growing number of people who will become HIV positive and develop AIDS-related illnesses. HIV epidemics in Eastern Europe and southeast Asia, while not as large as those in southern Africa, are among the fastest growing in the world. For example, the number of people living with HIV in Vietnam more than doubled between 2000 and 2005, and Ukraine has seen the number of new annual cases of HIV double since 2001.[9]

Whatever the HIV prevalence rate is, it does not reflect the full burden that HIV/AIDS inflicts on communities and entire nations. As prevalence rates estimate only the percentage of individuals currently infected, they do not take into account people who have already died and those who are likely to become infected. For example, it has been estimated that over half of the fifteen-year-old boys in Zimbabwe will die of AIDS if there is no change in the current trends.[10] The global AIDS epidemic has been identified by the United Nations Development Program as having inflicted in recent decades "the single greatest reversal in human development."[11]

Why Prevention Is Important

The old adage that "an ounce of prevention is worth a pound of cure" is the foundation of any sound public health policy. And HIV is, to use the memorable phrase of Cambridge epidemiologist Daniel Low-Beer, "a routinely avoidable disease."[12] HIV/AIDS is a chronic condition; it brings much suffering and is ultimately fatal. The humanitarian imperative for reducing this kind of physical suffering is further strengthened by the intense emotional fallout and anguish that often accompany infection with HIV and AIDS. An infected person may often experience psychological and emotional trauma, or face stigma and other forms of alienation.

Advocating the best means of avoiding HIV—to spare people these miseries, physical suffering, and death—remains an eminently humane priority. Prevention of HIV transmission takes on added urgency in parts of the world such as Africa where the epidemic is often generalized, treatment is limited, and consequences of infection are so severe and wide-ranging.

Besides the mortality and decreased life expectancy, prevention of further HIV transmission remains urgent for many other reasons. The epidemic has strained the ability of families and communities to care for those who are sick or orphaned; according to UNAIDS, in 2005 there were an estimated twelve million AIDS orphans in sub-Saharan Africa alone.[13] The epidemic has severely damaged social structures and weakened economic productivity. HIV/AIDS "generates new poverty" by leading to reductions in income as well as a depreciation of various human, physical, and social assets.[14] Effective prevention would also lead to fewer cases of mother-to-child transmission.[15]

Even with the recently expanded provision of antiretroviral therapy in developing nations, six new people are infected for every one who gets treatment. Despite global treatment targets, it remains unclear how financing for lifelong antiretroviral therapy can be sustained, given the accumulating number of new infections. And since infected people on treatment may feel more protected, let down their guard, and participate in risky behavior, there is the need to complement the expanding availability of antiretroviral therapy with redoubled efforts at prevention.[16] Thus, there are many evident rationales for more effective HIV prevention.

The Crisis in Prevention

Despite recent and welcome gains in international commitment and capacity to provide care and treatment for persons with HIV/AIDS in countries where such care has long been out of reach, we still face a crisis in preventing additional infections. The current efforts to provide care and treatment—advanced by generous initiatives such as PEPFAR (the President's Emergency Plan for AIDS Relief) and the Global Fund to Fight AIDS, Tuberculosis, and Malaria—were preceded by a lengthy period characterized almost exclusively by attempts to contain the further spread of HIV using risk reduction techniques. Yet an article in a 2003 issue of the *British Medical Journal* characterized the ensuing "rapid spread of HIV in sub-Saharan Africa"—despite our detailed knowledge of HIV epidemiology and the substantial investment in risk reduction—as "one of the greatest failures in the history of public health."[17]

The spread of HIV/AIDS and the impact of the various local and international responses are a complex matter which defies simple explanation. One thing, however, stands out: *the reluctance of the AIDS Establishment to encourage the avoidance of the behaviors that facilitate HIV transmission*. Resistance to "primary behavior change" was fierce in the initial stages of the international response. While this resistance has moderated recently, it still persists. Indeed, with few exceptions, the international response has focused on reducing the risks of acquiring HIV in already inherently risky behavior by encouraging condom use, voluntary counseling and testing, and the treatment of sexually transmitted infections.

These risk reduction interventions have been emphasized to such an extent that approaches that promote behaviors enabling people to avoid the risk of contracting the virus altogether are generally downplayed. Little attention and, until recently, almost no resources have been devoted to risk avoidance interventions such as abstinence and fidelity. (These behaviors, which constitute the A and B components of the ABC approach, are sometimes described in secularized terminology as "delaying sexual debut" and "partner reduction.")

Nevertheless, scientific evidence indicates that risk avoidance is what is most desperately needed to reverse the HIV/AIDS epidemic. Some real progress, however, has been made in recent years to increase the role of A and B interventions, notably through the efforts of many fair-minded scientists in the medical and research community and through the generous financial commitments of PEPFAR.

Notes

1. Centers for Disease Control and Prevention, *HIV and Its Transmission*, fact sheet, July 1999, http://www.cdc.gov/hiv/resources/factsheets/PDF/ transmission.pdf.

2. Helen Epstein, "Africa's Lethal Web Net of AIDS: The Quiet Acceptance of Informal Polygamy Is Spreading the Risk," *Los Angeles Times*, April 15, 2007, http:// articles.latimes.com/2007/apr/15/opinion/op-epstein15.

3. Daniel T. Halperin et al., "The Time Has Come for Common Ground on Preventing Sexual Transmission of HIV," *Lancet* 364.9449 (November 27–December 3, 2004): 1913–1915.

4. Bertran Auvert et al., "Randomized, Controlled Intervention Trial of Male Circumcision for Reduction of HIV Infection

AFFIRMING LOVE, AVOIDING AIDS

Risk: The ANRS 1265 Trial," *PLoS Medicine* 2.11 (November 2005): 1112–1122; Ronald H. Gray et al., "Male Circumcision for HIV Prevention in Men in Rakai, Uganda: A Randomised Trial," *Lancet* 369.9562 (February 24, 2007): 657; and Robert C. Bailey et al., "Male Circumcision for HIV Prevention in Young Men in Kisumu, Kenya: A Randomized Controlled Trial," *Lancet* 369.9562 (February 24, 2007): 643–656.

5. Alan D. Lopez et al., "Global and Regional Burden of Disease and Risk Factors, 2001: Systematic Analysis of Population Health Data," *Lancet* 367.9524 (May 27, 2006): 1747–1757.

6. Joint U.N. Programme on HIV/AIDS and World Health Organization, *AIDS Epidemic Update: December 2007* (UNAIDS/07.27E), http://data.unaids.org/pub/EPISlides/2007/2007_epi update_en.pdf.

7. U.N. Development Program, *Human Development Report 2005: International Cooperation at a Crossroads—Air, Trade and Security in an Unequal World* (New York: UNDP, 2005), http://hdr.undp.org/en/media/HDR05_complete.pdf.

8. Laurie Garrett, "The Lessons of HIV/AIDS," *Foreign Affairs* 84.4 (July–August 2005): 51–64.

9. "Status of the Global HIV Epidemic," chapter 2 of UNAIDS, *2008 Report on the Global AIDS Epidemic,* Geneva,August 2008, 48 and 52, http://data.unaids.org/pub/GlobalReport/2008/jc1510_2008_global_report_pp29_62 _en.pdf.

10. U.S. Agency for International Development, *The ABCs of HIV Prevention: Report of the USAID Technical Meeting on Behavior Change Approaches to Primary Prevention of HIV/AIDS*, Washington, D.C., September 17, 2002, http://www.usaid .gov/our_work/global_health/aids/TechAreas/prevention/abc. pdf.

11. UNDP, *Human Development Report 2005*.

12. Daniel Low-Beer, "Going Face to Face with AIDS: This Is a Routinely Avoidable Disease," *Financial Times*, November 28, 2003.

13. "Overview of the Global AIDS Epidemic," chapter 2 of UNAIDS, *2006 Report on the Global AIDS Epidemic*, Geneva, May 2006, 15, http://data.unaids.org/pub/GlobalReport/2006/2006 _GR_CH02_en.pdf.

14. Winford Masanjala, "The Poverty-HIV/AIDS Nexus in Africa: A Livelihood Approach," *Social Science and Medicine* 64.5 (March 2007): 1032–1041.

15. Centers for Disease Control and Prevention, "Achievements in Public Health: Reduction in Perinatal Transmission of HIV Infection—United States, 1985–2005," *Morbidity and Mortality Weekly Report* 55.21 (June 2, 2006): 592–597.

16. Waimar Tun et al., "Attitudes toward HIV Treatments Influence Unsafe Sexual and Injection Practices among Injecting Drug Users," *AIDS* 17.13 (September 5, 2003): 1953–1962.

17. Malcolm Potts and Julia Walsh, "Tackling India's HIV Epidemic: Lessons from Africa," *British Medical Journal* 326.7403 (June 21, 2003): 1389–1392.

III

ABSTINENCE AND FIDELITY

In December 2004, an international consensus on the ABC strategy for HIV prevention was published in the British medical journal *Lancet*.[1] A turning point in HIV/AIDS prevention, this consensus was signed by one-hundred forty people from thirty-six countries on the various continents. Fifty were professors and researchers at top universities (including Cambridge, Harvard, and Johns Hopkins universities, the Universities of California at Berkeley, Paris, and Brussels, and the London School of Hygiene and Tropical Medicine), and five were members of U.N. agencies. It was also signed by the director of the World Health Organization's HIV/AIDS programs and leaders of the HIV/AIDS programs of various countries worldwide, including Ethiopia, India, Jamaica, and Uganda.

It laid out in technical terms their rationale for prioritizing A, B, and C for different age groups, populations, and scenarios. In many respects, it amounted to a breakthrough—to a belated endorsement of A and B, which in years past would have been unthinkable. Since then, however, there have been many instances of reverting to business as usual, with an overwhelming bias in favor of condom promotion.

Are Abstinence and Fidelity Possible?

Edward C. Green and Allison Herling of Harvard University's AIDS Prevention Research Project, among other researchers, have provided convincing answers to the common criticisms of promoting abstinence and fidelity, such as criticism that it is not realistic, it promotes stigma, and it does not protect women.[2] Here we will address one central question: Is behavioral change in A and B possible, that is, are abstinence and fidelity practicable goals?

The best biological and survey data show that for the majority of Africans abstinence and fidelity are possible.[3] Data for 2001 from twenty-two sub-Saharan countries show that the majority of males and females aged fifteen to twenty-four years did not report premarital sex. In fact, more than 60 percent of females did not report premarital sex in sixteen of the twenty-two countries, while more than 50 percent of males did not report premarital sex in fifteen of these countries. So we cannot say that premarital sex is the norm for Africa.

Similar data from fifteen sub-Saharan African countries show that from 92 to 99 percent of sexually active females in all fifteen countries did not report multiple partners. Even for males, in thirteen of the fifteen countries more than 70 percent did not report multiple sexual partners. Infidelity in marriage is also not the norm for the vast majority of Africans. Data from the United Nations Population Division also indicate that limiting sexual activity to one partner is the most common behavioral change for people facing the threat of HIV/AIDS, whether in Africa, Asia, or Latin America.[4]

These data provide overwhelming evidence that premarital abstinence and fidelity in marriage are the norm for the vast majority of Africans.[5] They suggest that donors, international health organizations, and even many of the communities themselves need to expand their understanding of which behaviors are realistic and which interventions are feasible.

By way of comparison, it once seemed "unrealistic" to combat tobacco use when more than 75 percent of the population in many age groups smoked. But recognizing the serious health risks of tobacco use, public health authorities did not encourage people to smoke cigarettes with filters to reduce the risk of disease; rather, they encouraged people not to start smoking and to give up smoking if they were smokers. It is noteworthy that public health entities seek to modify some lifestyle choices but not others. The consumption of tobacco, cholesterol-laden diets, sedentary lifestyles, and reckless driving are all considered behaviors that require modification, but sexual behavior associated with disease and other adverse consequences is not.

Thirteen years before the 2004 *Lancet* consensus, representatives from several African countries met prior to an international AIDS conference held in Dakar, Senegal, in December 1991. They drew up a "statement of belief" about the centrality and feasibility of behavioral change in overcoming the AIDS epidemic. They declared,

> We believe that individuals and whole communities have the inherent capacity to change attitudes and behavior. The power to fulfill this capacity is often denied or is not exercised. This power must now be recognized, called forth and supported from both within and without. This will enable people to initiate, change and sustain behavior that promotes a healthy state of mind, body, spirit and environment. A critical component in this process is a supportive response to those living with HIV in the community.
>
> We recognize that behavior change at individual and community level in the present HIV pandemic is a complex and ongoing process. It is inextricably linked to such basic human values as care, love, faith, family and friendship, respect for people and cultures, solidarity and support. The present pandemic affects everyone. Our experience as affected and infected individuals proves that behavior change is possible. We believe that behavior change is the most essential strategy in overcoming the HIV pandemic.[6]

The International AIDS Society, which hosts these biennial international AIDS conferences, did not wish to accommodate this belief system. These African representatives were thus sidelined in their efforts to advance this concept during the conference. However, the data indicate that their beliefs were well founded.

Well over a decade later, Ugandan president Yoweri Museveni addressed the 2004 International AIDS conference held in Bangkok. Activists generated international headlines by denouncing him for his A- and B-oriented approach to HIV prevention. Given that Uganda has had by far the greatest success the world has seen in reducing its HIV prevalence, such protest was not only misplaced but unseemly.

The Urgent Need for Abstinence and Fidelity

An explanation of how multiple and concurrent partnerships can be so dangerous will show the urgency of focusing on A and B. Trying to understand the patterns of interpersonal connection and transmission, researchers from the University of Pennsylvania observed the inhabitants of seven villages on an island in Lake Malawi. They found that two-thirds of the inhabitants of the island were linked together by a single chain of sexual relationships over the three-year study period. In the journal *AIDS*, they went on to note that in such environments, "there are thus several potential paths between any two individuals in a network, rather than just one."[7]

Even though most individuals may not have a large number of partners, because so many people have multiple partners, a dense network of connectivity is created through which HIV is more readily transmitted. Indeed, someone with only one partner may be connected to a much larger network through that partner and thus be at a substantially elevated risk. In such a network structure, the chances that even a weakened virus will spread and infect a major proportion of the population remain high.[8]

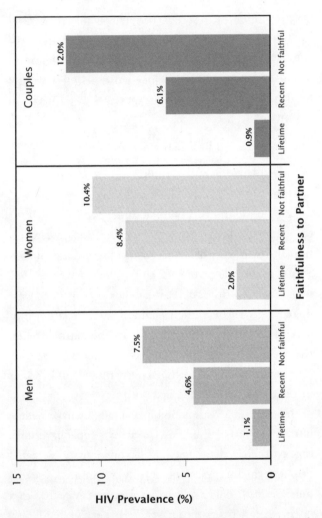

Figure 1. HIV prevalence by partner faithfulness. This graph shows the association between greater faithfulness and lower prevalence of HIV, based on data from Cameroon collected between 2004 and 2006. *Lifetime faithfulness* indicates persons

Communities in which people are able to modify this pattern and reduce multiple partnerships weaken the network and interrupt HIV transmission to a significant degree (Figure 1). This provides a compelling rationale for emphasizing risk avoidance messages in responses to HIV/AIDS.

Formidable epidemiological evidence from Africa further demonstrates the indispensable role that behavior has played in practice. Fundamental changes in "primary"

---

or couples who report never having had sex with anyone other than their current partner, and *recent faithfulness* indicates those with multiple lifetime sexual partners but no outside partners in the last twelve months; *not faithful* indicates those with multiple lifetime sexual partners and one or more outside partners in the last twelve months. For couples, mutual faithfulness is similarly defined, and HIV prevalence indicates that one or both partners were infected. Vinod Mishra and coworkers conclude that "having fewer lifetime sexual partners and being faithful to spousal partner(s) are strongly associated with reduced risk of HIV infection. Thus ... HIV prevention programs should focus more on promoting partner reduction and partner faithfulness, especially for men." Source: David Stanton, presented by Daniel Halperin in "Why Is HIV Prevalence So High in Southern Africa, and What Can Be Done about It?" Harvard Medical School, Boston, June 17, 2008, slide 31, based on data from Vinod Mishra et al., *The Role of Partner Reduction and Faithfulness in HIV Prevention in Sub-Saharan Africa: Evidence from Cameroon, Rwanda, Uganda, and Zimbabwe*, DHS working paper 61, Macro International for USAID, January 2009, 10, http://www.measuredhs.com/pubs/pdf/WP61/WP61.pdf.

sexual behavior are always found when HIV/AIDS prevalence declines.[9] Indeed, every instance in which HIV rates have fallen in Africa is most attributable to fundamental changes in sexual behavior—particularly declines in multiple sexual partnerships.

David Wilson, who monitors HIV/AIDS trends for the World Bank, observed that successful responses have typically been created and developed locally (often without the assistance of specialist agencies), have transformed norms of sexual behavior in the community, and have triggered rapid changes in behaviors and, therefore, in the incidence of the disease.[10]

Cambridge scholar Daniel Low-Beer observes that when this was not done, "HIV did not decline, even with greater resources, condom use, counseling, education, and treatment."[11] There is, therefore, a broad empirical and epidemiological rationale for emphasizing strategies A and B—abstinence and fidelity—for HIV prevention. We must apply these lessons to reverse the AIDS epidemic.[12]

The most well-known and most dramatic example of success comes from Uganda, where the HIV infection rate dropped from 15 percent in 1991 to 5 percent in 2001.[13] This decrease was "unique in the world" and "no other country has matched this achievement—at least not nationally," UNAIDS declared in its 2003 *AIDS Epidemic Update* report, which, curiously, provided no additional details.[14] In the five-year period during which Uganda achieved an 80 percent decrease in its HIV incidence, the country spent the modest sum of just twenty-one million dollars.[15] In fact, the behavioral changes were roughly equivalent to an 80 percent effective "social vaccine," one that was considerably more effective than any measure available now or conceivable in the near future, such as a vaccine or microbicides, and immeasurably less expensive.

What had happened there? The short answer is that profound shifts in actual sexual behavior, particularly increases in abstinence and fidelity, led to many fewer new cases of HIV transmission. This wholly rational decision to avoid the risk of a fatal and traumatic disease by altering behavior ultimately spared millions of lives.

The reduction in the number of sexual partners was the most significant factor in reducing HIV/AIDS incidence,[16] with an estimated decrease of 65 percent between 1989 and 1995 in the number of people who said they had sporadic sexual relations.[17] The adoption of risk avoidance behaviors was so thorough in Uganda that by the mid-1990s, 95 percent of adults said they had only one partner or none at all.[18] The percentage of men who said they had more than three partners decreased from 15 to 3 percent, significantly lower than the percentage in Cameroon, Zambia, and Kenya.[19] In 1989, the number of "non-regular" partners reported in Uganda was similar to the numbers in Kenya, Zambia, and Malawi. By the mid-1990s, however, it was 60 percent lower in Uganda than in these countries (Figure 2, *next page*).[20] While the rate of condom use in Uganda was similar to that in Zambia, Kenya, and Malawi in the mid-1990s, the percentage of

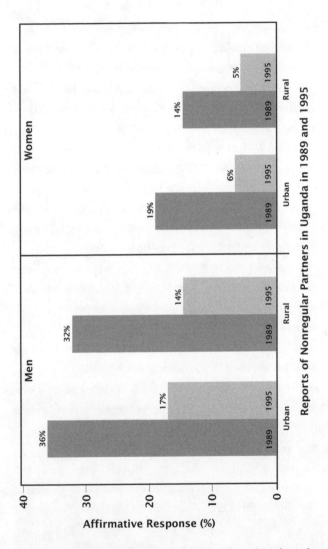

FIGURE 2. Behavioral change in Uganda. These data show the substantial reduction from 1989 to 1995 in the percentage of men and women reporting one or more non-regular (casual)

people in Uganda with multiple sexual partners was notably lower.[21] This difference largely explains the decrease
in the HIV rate in Uganda and the lack of a decrease in
Kenya, Zambia, and Malawi.

The evidence also reveals that abstinence contributed
to the decline. The percentage of young people who post-
poned the start of sexual relations increased, and virginity
among Ugandans between the ages of fifteen and nineteen
years increased significantly. There was also a pronounced
decrease in sporadic sexual relations. In the mid-1990s,
only 9 percent of single Ugandan women between the
ages of fifteen and twenty-four years said they had had a
sexual partner in the past year.[22]

Uganda was able to reduce its HIV rate before the
expansion of social marketing of condoms and voluntary
counseling and testing services. The social marketing of
condoms refers to the strategy condom companies employ
to create demand for their product, appealing to as wide

---

sexual partners in the past year. The overall reduction was 60
percent. Stoneburner and Low-Beer note that "the Ugandan
approach to HIV control was practical but based on limited
information, financial resources, and precedent for success. The
government communicated a clear warning and prevention
recommendation: AIDS ... was fatal and required an immediate population response based on ... faithfulness to one
partner." SOURCE: Graph adapted from Rand L. Stoneburner
and Daniel Low-Beer, "Population-Level HIV Declines and
Behavioral Risk Avoidance in Uganda," *Science* 304.5671
(April 30, 2004), 716.

a population as possible, if not to the masses. Voluntary counseling and testing refers to the practice of promoting testing and counseling services to people who suspect they may have HIV or may have been exposed to it. Voluntary counseling and testing programs rely heavily on condom promotion.

In 1989, fewer than 3 percent of Ugandan women had reported ever using condoms. By 1995, that figure was still less than 8 percent—the lowest of the countries in that region. These low figures stand out against the fact that African countries with the highest availability of condoms also have some of the highest HIV/AIDS rates in the world.[23] These countries include Botswana, Zimbabwe, and South Africa.

Uganda's response included educational sessions in schools and the empowerment and training of women and young people to take responsibility for their own health. The involvement of religious leaders and the leadership of President Museveni facilitated this response. They emphasized a change in traditional relationships between men and women, which meant defending chaste behavior in the sense of "sexual abstinence before marriage and mutual fidelity within marriage," and reestablishing these behaviors as valued social norms. Speaking to an international AIDS conference, Museveni said,

> In the olden days you offered us the magic bullet of penicillin, now we are being told to protect our lives by a mere bit of rubber. In a country like mine where people have to walk five kilometers to get an aspirin,

do you think that they will go there to get a condom?
That is why I am asking my people to go back to our
time-tested culture of no premarital sex and faithfulness
in marriage. Young people need to be taught discipline,
self-control, and at times sacrifice.[24]

Catholic nuns and doctors, active at the grass roots
in providing medical care to those who live with AIDS,
developed their own process for behavioral change.
Known as "Education for Life" or "Youth Alive," it holds
as a defining principle that people can control and change
their behavior. Workshops facilitating responsible choices
and behavior change were carried out in schools, parishes,
and other institutes. Youth Alive clubs were established
to provide follow-up character formation and to transform peer pressure. The program has been exported from
Uganda to several other African countries and used with
positive results.[25]

Meanwhile, the role of religious leaders in combating HIV/AIDS cannot be underestimated. In Uganda,
for example, an Anglican bishop and a Catholic bishop
were among the first presidents of the country's AIDS
commission.[26] Entire reports describe the constructive,
if relatively untapped, role of faith-based organizations
in HIV prevention around the world.[27]

Rand Stoneburner of Cambridge University estimated
that if a Uganda-style ABC program had been implemented in Africa in 1996, through 2004 six million new
infections would have been averted and four million fewer
children would have been orphaned.[28] This suggests that

failure to support these interventions has had devastating consequences.

Indeed, there is evidence of such failure to emphasize A and B interventions even in Uganda itself. Despite their initial and unparalleled success, Uganda's own locally derived methods for facing the threat of HIV gradually gave way to the demands and priorities of foreign donor agencies and allegedly nongovernmental organizations. No longer did Uganda resist the Western emphasis on condoms. Billboards with messages about condoms began to replace those which formerly promoted abstinence and fidelity. The director of Harvard's AIDS Prevention Research Project, Edward C. Green, writes that "during a meeting of top religious leaders in Uganda in November 2004, one cleric after another complained that they had become increasingly marginalized, while foreign experts scoffed at abstinence and faithfulness as prevention strategies."[29] We can also attest to the accuracy of that statement from personal experience, having addressed more than one hundred Catholic bishops from eight African countries in Uganda in 2005.

Sam Ruteikara, the co-chair of Uganda's National AIDS Prevention Committee, bemoaned the AIDS Establishment's harmful influence in a 2008 *Washington Post* piece, writing that AIDS "has become a multibillion-dollar industry," in which profiteering (from the sale of commodities such as condoms and test kits) and ideology have supplanted sound approaches to prevention.[30]

That may sound like a serious charge, but it is difficult to dismiss given Ruteikara's exasperating personal experience with Western donor agencies, which systematically resisted the inclusion of abstinence and fidelity messages in national strategic plans and removed them when they did appear, even though his country's unparalleled success in reducing AIDS transmission was due to those components in the first place.[31]

In fact, AIDS prevalence has gone back *up* in recent years as the focus has shifted away from Uganda's original emphasis on fidelity and toward the international donor emphasis on condoms, even though this increase is often depicted in the press as stemming from not enough condoms. National survey data from 2004 confirmed an increase in the level of multiple partnerships and an HIV prevalence rate which had increased to 7 percent.[32]

Thailand offers another example of success. Although its decision to emphasize mandatory condom use in commercial sex establishments is reflexively credited with causing a decline in HIV prevalence, more fundamental shifts in behavioral patterns have also contributed greatly to the decline. Between 1990 and 1993, the percentage of men who had relations with commercial sex workers decreased by more than half (from 22 to 10 percent). The proportion of men who said that in the preceding year they had had sexual relations outside a relationship with a stable partner dropped from 28 to 15 percent.[33] These declines, as well as the fact that commercial sex workers were the last group to show declines in HIV, suggest that this risk avoidance was "at least as important as increase in condom use."[34] Furthermore, other sexually transmitted infections that are transmitted "skin to skin" also declined, and condom use does not typically protect against such infections.[35] Finally, the fact that women had very low rates of sexual relations outside a relationship with a stable partner[36] played a key role in preventing the expansion of HIV transmission.

There are encouraging trends and successful examples of behavior change and declining prevalence in other African countries besides Uganda, such as Kenya and Zimbabwe, and in Haiti, the country with the most severe epidemic outside Africa. The data from Kenya appears to be the strongest. Since the late 1990s, the HIV rate has sharply declined in many parts of the country, triggered by significant behavior change.[37] Between 1998 and 2003, the percentage of unmarried people who reported having had no sex in the past year increased significantly and the percentage of men and women who reported having two or more partners in the past year declined about 50 percent. Those reporting two or more partners in the past year were twice as likely to be infected with HIV as those reporting one partner. There was little change in condom use in this period. Due to these increases in abstinence and faithfulness (A and B), HIV prevalence in Kenya dropped from 9.4 percent in 1998 to 6.7 percent in 2003.[38]

For quite some time, Zimbabwe emphasized condom use (C), but to no avail. Along with Botswana, Swaziland,

and South Africa, Zimbabwe had one of the most severe epidemics anywhere. Recent empirical data published in the journal *Science,* however, indicate that behavior has changed, and as a result HIV prevalence has also decreased there.[39] While it continues to have one of the highest prevalence rates in the world, the rate has fallen from over 32 percent in 2000 to approximately 24 percent in 2004. While condom use with casual partners remained stable among men (41.6 percent in 1998–2000 and 42.2 percent in 2001–2003) and increased among women (from 26.2 to 36.5 percent in the same period), more significant changes in sexuality were observed in the population.[40]

The percentage of young people postponing sexual activity increased and that of young adults (aged fifteen to twenty-nine years) having multiple partners markedly decreased.[41] The percentage of men aged fifteen to seventeen years who said they had already started having sexual relations dropped from 45 percent between 1998 and 2000 to 27 percent between 2001 and 2003. Among women, this figure fell from 21 to 9 percent. Among people who were sexually active, the percentage of men who said they had casual sexual relations dropped from 25.9 to 13.2 percent. In both sexes, there was a statistically significant decrease in the number of new sexual partners during the year prior to the survey, in the number of sexual partners during the preceding month, and in current sexual partners.[42] It appears that the most influential factors in lowering the prevalence rate were the increase in the age at which adolescent men and women began having sexual relations and the decrease in the number of casual sexual partners among those who were already sexually active.

Haiti's estimated HIV prevalence in 2000 was 5.5 percent, the highest in the Western hemisphere—indeed anywhere outside of Africa. It has since fallen to 3 percent. This significant decline was also preceded by and attributable to an increase in B-related behaviors—that is, in fidelity. Rigorous mathematical modeling published in the journal *Sexually Transmitted Infections* indicated that the decline in the HIV prevalence rate in Kenya, Zimbabwe, and Haiti was due not to the natural course of an epidemic but to changes in sexual behavior.[43] This is an important point, for although some have argued that reductions in AIDS rates resulted from the artificial effect of greater mortality among infected persons rather than from a real decrease in new cases of infection, the most important factor in these countries was an increase in fidelity and a reduction in sexual partnering.[44] Indeed, these fundamental changes in sexual behavior are responsible for declines in generalized epidemics as well as concentrated epidemics.[45]

There are encouraging signs from other countries as well. In Rwanda, a "unique combination of low numbers of partners and late sexual debut" has helped forestall an larger epidemic.[46] In Malawi, survey data suggest at least some declines in HIV incidence and prevalence.[47] In Ethiopia, there were significant declines in the late 1990s in the proportion of male factory workers around Addis Ababa engaging in casual sex and in sex with commercial sex workers.[48] HIV prevalence among women at antenatal clinics in Addis Ababa dropped from 18.2 percent in 1997 to 11.8 percent in 2003.[49] Prevalence among those seeking counseling and testing at two sites in Addis Ababa declined from 29 to 15 percent between 2002 and 2004, and these declines were associated with declines in risky behavior, notably a decline in casual sexual contacts.[50] For youth aged fifteen to twenty-four years, the decline was even steeper: from 22 percent in 2002 to 9 percent in 2004. Condom use did not increase, and in fact the proportion of clients aged twenty-five to forty-nine who reported never using a condom increased somewhat.[51]

In contrast with the African countries that have achieved a reversal in their epidemics, South Africa's persistent rates of multiple partnerships have helped maintain its sustained, alarmingly high incidence.[52] South African anthropologist Suzanne Leclerc-Madlala, lamenting her country's ongoing and devastating HIV rate, characterized the national prevention approach as having gone "straight for the C option and [placing] little emphasis on A and B."[53] She wrote that South Africans have been reluctant "to accept the idea that [the spread of AIDS] has much to do with sexual responsibility" and that "our hip-hyped AIDS prevention campaign and its condom-promoting 'have fun but play safely' message has thus far failed us as a people." Abstinence and fidelity are unpopular, she continued, and

> there are many fears to be faced in this epidemic, and some of them have to do with our fear of taking an

41

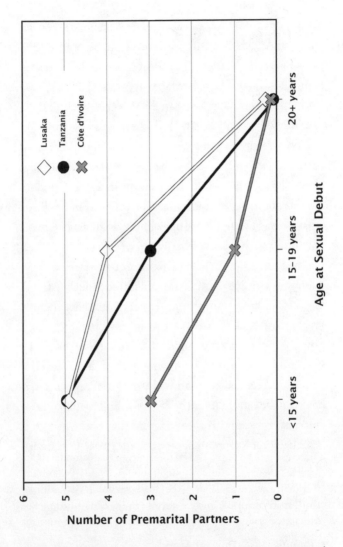

FIGURE 3. Number of premarital partners by age at sexual debut. These 2001 data show the positive relationship between later age at first intercourse and fewer premarital sexual partners

unpopular stand, of being associated with the moral right, or of being labeled a "this" or a "that." In our current context, abstinence and faithfulness are simply the "safest-sex" messages that we have. Why then have these messages not been given a fraction of the media time and attention that we have given to the promotion of condoms?[54]

While fidelity (B) appears to have been the most important factor in Africa's successes, abstinence (A) is also important—both for the young and for many others, such as widows. Abstinence influences future behavior. For instance, the earlier a person initiates sexual activity, the more lifetime sexual partners that person is likely to have, thus increasing the person's risk of contracting HIV and other sexually transmitted infections (Figure 3, *opposite*, and Figure 4, *next page*).[55] These are other findings of note:

- Some types of human papillomavirus tend to become chronic and lead to genital cancer,[56] and the

---

among men in Lusaka, Tanzania, and Côte d'Ivoire. Partner reduction is the most vital epidemiological variable, and it rightly deserves far greater emphasis. But it should not be forgotten that abstinence also often helps shape later behavior. It is thus important for its own sake and for its role in limiting future sexual contacts. SOURCE: Population, Health and Nutrition Information Project, *The ABCs of HIV Prevention: Report of a USAID Technical Meeting on Behavior Change Approaches to Primary Prevention of HIV/AIDS*, USAID, September 17, 2002, page 6, based on data from a USAID report of November 16, 2001.

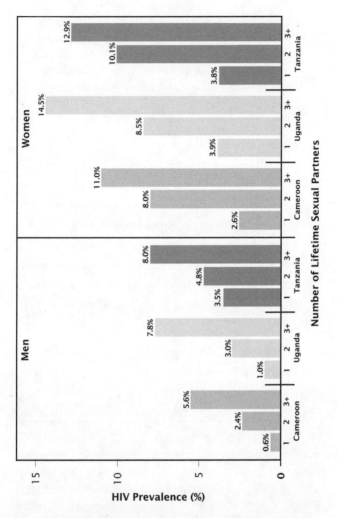

FIGURE 4. HIV prevalence by number of lifetime sexual partners. These data from Cameroon, Uganda, and Tanzania show that HIV prevalence increases with the number of sexual partners. Responding more intelligently and honestly to the

younger a person is when infected, the greater the risk that the infection could develop into cancer.

- The frequency of disappointment with and regret about having had an early sexual encounter is inversely proportional to the person's age at the time of sexual initiation.[57]

- Preventive health education programs that focus on sexual behavior are less effective among people who began having sexual relations at an early age.[58]

- Although cervical secretions provide protection against bacteria and viruses,[59] because of the relative immaturity of the cervix in adolescent women, they are considerably less protected than adult women.

An extensive USAID multi-country study, which looked at the variables associated with HIV prevalence in four African nations (Benin, Cameroon, Kenya, and Zambia) representing each of the regions of the continent, yielded important but unanticipated results. It concluded that the only factors significantly associated with lower HIV prevalence were lower lifetime number of partners (fidelity), an older age of sexual debut (abstinence), and

------

AIDS epidemic requires moving beyond technically oriented risk reduction strategies and grappling with the behavior that drives it. SOURCE: David Stanton, presented by Daniel Halperin in "Why Is HIV Prevalence So High in Southern Africa," slide 30, based on data from Vinod Mishra.

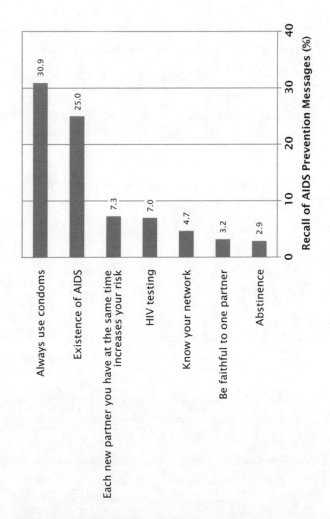

FIGURE 5. Recall of HIV prevention messages. This graph shows how commonly HIV prevention messages were recalled by Basotho men in Lesotho in 2009. The messages were received largely from radio, television, and print sources. The most commonly recalled messages were about condom usage and

male circumcision.[60] It also found that variables such as socio-economic status and condom use were not associated with lower HIV prevalence and that the presence of bacterial sexually transmitted infections was not predictive of HIV prevalence.

The overall evidence to date has prompted Leclerc-Madlala to conclude that

> If we are serious about slowing the growth of HIV in our population we need to be thinking of better ways to promote modifications in sexual behavior; programs aimed at interrupting the HIV transmission "engine" of concurrent sexual partnerships would likely have a great impact on slowing our local epidemic. There is a huge need for such programs, yet all we hear about is the need for better access to condoms.[61]

Survey data from Lesotho bring Leclerc-Madlala's observation into sharp relief (Figure 5). When a representative sample of Basotho men were asked to name prevention messages they could recall hearing about (from a variety of sources), respondents identified condoms far

---

general awareness of AIDS, while the men recalled relatively few messages about faithfulness and abstinence. Considering that condoms have not reduced generalized African epidemics, while changes in behavior have resulted in HIV reductions elsewhere in Africa, these data provide further indication of the need for public health initiatives to place greater emphasis on behavior change. SOURCE: Andy Tan et al. for USAID, *A Baseline Survey of Multiple and Concurrent Sexual Partnerships among Basotho Men in Lesotho*, C-Change/Academy for Educational Development, July 2009, 25.

more often than anything else. Abstinence and faithfulness were much less commonly recalled. In fact, the recall of condom messages exceeded the recall of both abstinence and faithfulness messages by approximately ten-fold each.

A recent *British Medical Journal* article also called for a renewed prioritization to change sexual behavior. The article included an appeal to the "common good" (generally rare in scientific publications dealing with matters of sexuality) and concluded that "we can help foster and reinforce shared perceptions that certain risk behaviors are both personally unwise and raise the burden and effects of disease for all."[62]

Other highly relevant studies, published in the *American Journal of Obstetrics and Gynecology* and the *African Journal of AIDS Research*, have called for the modification of the standard risk reduction approaches to sexually transmitted infections, and for authorities to respond more intelligently to epidemiological trends.[63] Inasmuch as how we define or diagnose a problem shapes how we will try to solve it, honesty about the behaviors and attitudes that drive HIV transmission is essential.

Notes

1. Daniel T. Halperin et al., "The Time Has Come for Common Ground on Preventing Sexual Transmission of HIV," *Lancet* 364.9449 (November 27, 2004): 1913–1915.

2. Edward C. Green and Allison Herling, *The ABC Approach to Preventing the Sexual Transmission of AIDS: Common*

Questions and Answers (Washington, D.C.: Christian Connections for International Health, February 2007), 44, http://www.harvardaidsprp.org/research/Green&Herling_ABC_Approach_Feb07(2).pdf.

3. M. Mahy and N. Gupta, "Trends and Differentials in Adolescent Reproductive Behavior in Sub-Saharan Africa," in *DHS Analytical Studies 3*, ed. Macro International and Measure DHS (Calverton, MD: ORC Macro, 2002).

4. U.N. Population Division, *HIV/AIDS Awareness and Behaviour* (ST/ESA/SER.A/209), 2002, http://www.un.org/esa/population/publications/AIDS_awareness/AIDS_English.pdf.

5. Mahy and Gupta, "Trends and Differentials."

6. This statement of belief can be found in "Combating the Spread of AIDS," by Sister Dr. Miriam Duggan, F.M.S.A., in *Culture of Life—Culture of Death*, ed. Luke Gormally (London: Linacre Center, 2002).

7. Stéphane Helleringer and Hans-Peter Kohler, "Sexual Network Structure and the Spread of HIV in Africa: Evidence from Likoma Island, Malawi," *AIDS* 21.17 (November 12, 2007): 2323–2332.

8. Ibid.

9. T. Stammers, "As Easy as ABC? Primary Prevention of Sexually Transmitted Infections," *Postgraduate Medicine Journal* 81.955 (May 2005): 273–275.

10. David Wilson, "Partner Reduction and the Prevention of HIV/AIDS," *British Medical Journal* 328.7444 (April 10, 2004): 848–849.

11. Daniel Low-Beer, "Going Face to Face with AIDS: This Is a Routinely Avoidable Disease," *Financial Times*, November 28, 2003.

12. Alvaro Alonso and Jokin de Irala, "Strategies in HIV Prevention: The A-B-C Approach," *Lancet* 364.9431 (July 24, 2004): 1033.

13. Janice A. Hogle, ed., *What Happened in Uganda? Declining HIV Prevalence, Behavior Change and the National Response* (Washington, D.C.: USAID, September 2002), http://www.usaid.gov/pop_health/aids/Countries/africa/uganda_report.pdf.

14. Joint U.N. Program on HIV/AIDS and World Health Organization, *AIDS Epidemic Update: December 2003* (UNAIDS/03.39E), 10, http://data.unaids.org/Publications/IRC-pub06/JC943-EpiUpdate2003_en.pdf.

15. Low-Beer, "Going Face to Face with AIDS."

16. See Edward C. Green, testimony before the U.S. Senate Subcommittee on Africa, May 19, 2003; and Edward C. Green et al., "Uganda's HIV Prevention Success: The Role of Sexual Behavior Change and the National Response," *AIDS Behavior* 10.4 (July 2006): 335–346.

17. Daniel Low-Beer and Rand L. Stoneburner, "Behavior and Communication Change in Reducing HIV: Is Uganda Unique?" *African Journal of AIDS Research* 2.1 (May 2003): 9–21.

18. Rand L. Stoneburner and Daniel Low-Beer, "Population-Level HIV Declines and Behavioral Risk Avoidance in Uganda," *Science* 304.5671 (April 30, 2004): 714–718.

19. Ruth Bessinger, Priscilla Akwara, and Daniel Halperin, *Sexual Behavior, HIV and Fertility Trends: A Comparative Analysis of Six Countries—Phase I of the ABC Study* (Washington, D.C.: USAID, 2003).

20. Population, Health and Nutrition Information Project, *The ABCs of HIV Prevention: Report of a USAID Technical Meeting*

on Behavior Change Approaches to Primary Prevention of HIV/ AIDS (Washington, D.C.: USAID, September 17, 2002), http://www.usaid.gov/our_work/global_health/aids/TechAreas/prevention/abc.pdf.

21. Ibid.

22. Ibid.

23. Edward C. Green, "Culture Clash and AIDS Prevention," *Responsive Community* 13.4 (2003): 4–9.

24. Yoweri Kaguta Museveni, "AIDS and Its Impact on the Health and Social Service and Infrastructure in Developing Countries," speech by the President of Uganda at the International Conference on AIDS, Florence, Italy, June 16, 1991.

25. Duggan, "Combating the Spread of AIDS."

26. Hogle, *What Happened in Uganda?*

27. Edward C. Green, *Faith-Based Organizations: Contributions to HIV Prevention* (Washington, D.C.: USAID and Synergy Project, September 2003); and Jeremy Liebowitz, *The Impact of Faith-Based Organizations on HIV/AIDS Prevention and Mitigation in Africa*, prepared for the Health Economics and HIV/AIDS Research Division, University of Natal, Durban, South Africa, October 2002, http://www.heard.org.za/heard -resources/assortment.

28. Patricia Thickstun and Kate Hendricks, eds., *Evidence That Demands Action: Comparing Risk Avoidance and Risk Reduction Strategies for HIV Prevention* (Austin, TX: Medical Institute for Sexual Health, 2004), iv, https://secure.digital -community.com/english/medinstitute.org/includes/down loads/abc.pdf?PHPSESSID=63bb6283d34c3a325166433 3d31acd74.

29. Edward C. Green, "AIDS in Africa—A Betrayal: The One Success Story Is Now Threatened by U.S. Aid Bureaucrats,"

Weekly Standard 10.19 (January 31, 2005), http://www.weekly standard.com/Content/Protected/Articles/000/000/005/172wwqzc.asp?pg=1.

30. Sam Ruteikara, "Let My People Go, AIDS Profiteers," *Washing-ton Post*, June 30, 2008, A11.

31. Matthew Hanley, "AIDS and 'Technical Solutions': First Change Sexual Behavior," *Ethics & Medics* 33.12 (December 2008): 1–3.

32. Green et al., "Uganda's HIV Prevention Success."

33. Low-Beer and Stoneburner, "Behavior and Communication Change."

34. Ibid.

35. Stephen J. Genuis and Shelagh K. Genuis, "Managing the Sexually Transmitted Disease Pandemic: A Time for Reevaluation," *American Journal of Obstetrics and Gynecology* 191.4 (October 2004): 1103–1112; and Rachel L. Winer et al., "Condom Use and the Risk of Genital Human Papillomavirus Infection in Young Women," *New England Journal of Medicine* 354.25 (June 22, 2006): 2645–2654.

36. PHNI Project, *ABCs of HIV Prevention.*

37. B. Cheluget et al., "Evidence for Population Level Declines in Adult HIV Prevalence in Kenya," *Sexually Transmitted Infections* 82, suppl. 1 (April 2006): i21–i26.

38. Edward C. Green, "ABC: Expanding Prevention Models to Generalized Epidemics," May 25, 2005, slide 62. See also the Kenya National AIDS/STD Control Program Web site at http://www.aidskenya.org.

39. Simon Gregson et al., "HIV Decline Associated with Behavior Change in Eastern Zimbabwe," *Science* 311.5761 (February 3, 2006): 664–666.

40. Green and Herling, *ABC Approach to Preventing*, 27–28.

41. A. Mahomva et al., "HIV Prevalence and Trends from Data in Zimbabwe: 1997–2004," *Sexually Transmitted Infections* 82, suppl. 1 (April 2006): i42–i47.

42. Gregson et al., "HIV Decline Associated with Behavior Change."

43. Timothy B. Hallett et al., "Declines in HIV Prevalence Can Be Associated with Changing Sexual Behaviour in Uganda, Urban Kenya, Zimbabwe, and Urban Haiti," *Sexually Transmitted Infections* 82, suppl. 1 (April 2006): i1–i8.

44. Southern African Development Community, *Expert Think Tank Meeting on HIV Prevention in High-Prevalence Countries in Southern Africa: Report*, Maseru, Lesotho, May 10–12, 2006 (Gaborone, Botswana: SADC, July 2006), http://data.unaids. org/pub/Report/2006/20060601_sadc_meeting_report _en.pdf.

45. Green and Herling, *ABC Approach to Preventing*, 28.

46. E. Kayirangwa et al., "Current Trends in Rwanda's HIV/ AIDS Epidemic," *Sexually Transmitted Infections* 82, suppl. 1 (April 2006): i27, http://www.ncbi.nlm.nih.gov/pmc/articles/ PMC2593071/pdf/i27.pdf.

47. G. A. Bello, J. Chipeta, and J. Aberle-Grasse, "Assessment of Trends in Biological and Behavioural Surveillance Data: Is There Any Evidence of Declining HIV Prevalence or Incidence in Malawi?" *Sexually Transmitted Infections* 82, suppl. 1 (April 2006): i9–i13.

48. Yared Mekonnen et al., "Evidence of Changes in Sexual Behavior among Male Factory Workers in Ethiopia," *AIDS* 17.2 (2003): 223–231.

49. Green and Herling, *ABC Approach to Preventing*, 29.

50. Ibid.

51. Ibid.

52. James D. Shelton, "Confessions of a Condom Lover," *Lancet* 368.9551 (December 2, 2006): 1947–1949.

53. See Suzanne Leclerc-Madlala, "Prevention Means More Than Condoms," *Mail and Guardian*, October 4, 2002, 19, http://www.aegis.com/news/dmg/2002/MG021003.html. We have also drawn on a lengthier, unpublished version of this article, obtained through correspondence with Leclerc-Madlala.

54. Ibid.

55. Genuis and Genuis, "Managing the Sexually Transmitted Disease Pandemic."

56. F. Xavier Bosch et al., "Epidemiology of Human Papillomavirus Infections and Associations with Cervical Cancer: New Opportunities for Prevention," in *Papillomavirus Research: From Natural History to Vaccines and Beyond*, ed. M. Saveria Campo (Wymondham, U.K.: Caister Academic, 2006).

57. Nigel Dickson et al., "First Sexual Intercourse: Age, Coercion, and Later Regrets Reported by a Birth Cohort," *British Medical Journal* 316.7124 (January 3, 1998): 29–33.

58. Jennifer K. Legardy et al., "Do Participant Characteristics Influence the Effectiveness of Behavioral Interventions? Promoting Condom Use to Women," *Sexually Transmitted Diseases* 32.11 (November 2005): 665–671.

59. Minnie John et al., "Cervicovaginal Secretions Contribute to Innate Resistance to Herpes Simplex Virus Infection," *Journal of Infectious Disease* 192.10 (2005): 1731–1740.

60. Bessinger, Akwara, and Halperin, *Sexual Behavior, HIV and Fertility Trends*, vii.

61. Suzanne Leclerc-Madlala, "The Behaviours and Beliefs That Are Driving AIDS Have to Change," *Sunday Independent* [South Africa], March 12, 2006, http://www.sunday independent.co.za/index.php.

62. Michael M. Cassell et al., "Risk Compensation: The Achilles' Heel of Innovations in HIV Prevention?" *British Medical Journal* 332.7541 (March 11, 2006): 605–607.

63. See, for example, Genuis and Genuis, "Managing the Sexually Transmitted Disease Pandemic," and Low-Beer and Stoneburner, "Behavior and Communication Change."

IV

The Failed
Public Health Response

"As AIDS educators," says David Wilson, "we often publicly promote approaches that we would not countenance in our own personal lives, such as the notion that it is acceptable for our spouses or our children to have multiple partners, provided condoms are used."[1]

Wilson's insight gets to the heart of the matter. It at once recognizes a universal ethical point of reference and demonstrates the AIDS Establishment's insistence on ignoring it. All persons long for love, respect, and fidelity —the very foundations of the Golden Rule, treating others as you would like them to treat you. The AIDS Establishment distances itself from this basic ethical norm. In place of the norm, they resolutely follow the imperative to appear nonjudgmental, approving of almost any form of behavior—as long as it is far removed from their own personal circumstances. The AIDS Establishment is committed to this viewpoint, even when it means turning a blind eye to contradictory or threatening data. Such a stance not only betrays considerable philosophical recklessness but also undermines its own scientific credibility.

Rejecting Abstinence and Fidelity Strategies

The AIDS Establishment has displayed a strong and consistent reluctance to acknowledge and act on evidence that shows the crucial role of behavioral change in slowing HIV transmission. In a 2003 *British Medical Journal* article, for example, Daniel Low-Beer explained that the declines in HIV resulting from a 65 percent decline in casual sex in Uganda were simply not described in UNAIDS reports.[2] The UNAIDS 2001 *Declaration of Commitment on HIV/AIDS* does state that "abstinence and fidelity" should be part of any comprehensive AIDS prevention program,[3] yet the UNAIDS 2005 *AIDS Epidemic Update* only refers to abstinence twice and to fidelity three times in the entire ninety-eight-page report. Neither word is mentioned favorably.[4]

Furthermore, when the 2005 *Epidemic Update* refers to the role played by abstinence and fidelity in decreasing HIV incidence and prevalence, it describes them ambiguously and even misleadingly. In referring to the decreases in Uganda and Kenya, for example, it states that "in both countries, behavioural changes are likely to have contributed to the trend shifts," leaving the reader unsure as to which behavioral changes it means and what effect they had.[5]

It also describes the condom as the most effective "technology" for AIDS prevention, overlooking the fact that the behavioral strategy of abstinence enables a person to avoid risk altogether, and ignoring the profound epidemiological impact partner reduction has had. Condoms might be the most effective "technology" for AIDS prevention, but they are certainly not the most effective prevention measure. Abstinence is the only 100 percent effective preventive measure; partner reduction is, of course, not the same as abstinence, or even comparable to lifelong monogamy or fidelity, yet it has proved to be a much more important factor than condoms in declines of HIV incidence.

A preparatory document for the 2005 World AIDS Day campaign includes a summary of the 2001 *Declaration of Commitment*, specifying among the goals of prevention efforts to "encourage responsible behaviour [and] expand access to male and female condoms."[6] Yet point 52 of the declaration originally spoke of "encouraging responsible sexual behaviour, *including abstinence and fidelity*; [and] expanded access to essential commodities, including male and female condoms."[7] Mention of abstinence and fidelity is wholly omitted from the 2005 summary.

In discussing Uganda's unparalleled success in reducing HIV prevalence for a 2005 PBS *NOW* documentary, UNAIDS executive director Peter Piot said, "The problem is of course that we will never know, probably, what percentage of the decline is due to condom use. What percentage is due to abstinence. And so ... you can't always disentangle that. But we also know that no country has been successful in bringing down the number of new infections of HIV without strong condom promotion."[8]

Never mind that Uganda's decline in HIV incidence could not possibly have been due to condom promotion, since the decline occurred well before Western donors flooded the country with condoms! Piot's statement only serves to obfuscate—to diminish the greatest contributions we described earlier: actual changes in primary behavior, measured in terms of greater levels of fidelity and of abstinence.

Furthermore, Piot's assertion here is almost diametrically opposed to global findings on declines in HIV prevalence: all the evidence indicates that the common denominator in HIV declines around the world is not the promotion of condoms but a reduction in sexual partners. Indeed, countries with the most robust condom promotion programs, such as South Africa, have some of the most severe AIDS epidemics in the world. Whatever the role of condoms may have been in averting some individual transmission in some settings, Piot's claim that condoms have been the universal key ingredient to declining rates of HIV infection is wildly misleading. While Piot's statements may both confirm and perpetuate the preconceptions of the AIDS Establishment, they have become increasingly hard to defend.

These examples are representative of the tendency to downplay or ignore abstinence and fidelity in official statements and reports.

Beneath the reluctance to promote abstinence and fidelity lies the assumption—at once patronizing and dangerous—that sexual behavior cannot be changed. At times this reluctance gives way to a militant conviction that, even in the face of HIV/AIDS, sexual behavior should not change. This explains the AIDS Establishment's overwhelming and reflexive recourse to technical "solutions."

This is not to say that people will respond to directives or prohibitions alone. Promoting risk avoidance is not without its challenges. What is needed is not simply information about disease but teaching that helps explain the deeper significance and meaning of sexuality and the dignity and respect due to every human being. Such an understanding makes clear the value of postponing the start of sexual relations and the value of mutually monogamous sexual relations. Interventions are needed to foster a greater understanding of sexuality and human dignity and to counter established norms that encourage behaviors which increase HIV transmission. The vision of sexuality that leads to behavior change is based on respect for oneself and for the other, and on hope for the future.[9] This broader context is particularly important since simply knowing about the risks of disease does not in itself lead to reductions in risky behaviors and disease prevalence.

There is also a need for strategies that foster healthy behaviors through social networks and community structures that influence individual behavior. The responsibility for transformation, therefore, does not rest solely on sexually active youth whose behavior places them at risk, for example, but also on older members of the community who, as guardians of the culture, uphold the dignity of every human person and the deeper understanding of sexuality.

It is not uncommon to hear that changing behavior, especially sexual behavior, will invariably take a long time. The AIDS Establishment offers this as an additional rationale for emphasizing technical rather than behavioral approaches to HIV prevention. As Wilson points out, however, one of the most striking but overlooked elements in the successful reductions of HIV prevalence is how quickly behavior changed, most notably in Uganda and Thailand.[10] This represents genuine cause for hope, for it shows that entire populations are capable of relatively rapid behavioral changes.

Thus, making risk avoidance a priority is not just a matter of investing resources but a matter of emphasis, of communicating commonsense ideas and of daring to uphold values and norms that run counter to those cherished by the AIDS Establishment.

Overselling Condom Effectiveness

While measuring the effectiveness of condoms in preventing HIV transmission is inherently difficult, the most detailed scientific estimates range from 80 to 90 percent. A 2000 study by the National Institutes of Health put the figure at about 85 percent, a 2003 UNAIDS review of literature on condoms in developing countries puts it at 90 percent, and a study published in the *Cochrane Review* puts it at 80 percent.[11] Since condom use with an infected partner carries a risk of infection, repeated exposure increases the likelihood of infection over time. Even with "perfect" condom use, HIV may eventually be transmitted.

But it is necessary to understand these data. Saying that condom use reduces risk by 80 percent does not mean "there is a 20 percent failure rate." When "discordant" couples (one person is infected and the other is not) have sexual relations over the course of a year without using a condom, the infection rate is about 5.7 percent. If they always use a condom, and use it correctly, this risk will be reduced by 80 percent, to a rate of 1.14 percent (5.7 x 0.8 = 4.56, and 5.7 − 4.56 = 1.14). This probability of infection tends to be lower when the infected person is receiving appropriate antiretroviral treatment, but it can be higher if that person is not on treatment—which is far too common in severe African epidemics. These results come from a review of 4,709 scientific bibliographic references and selected studies that allowed valid comparisons.[12]

Although with condom use the probability of HIV infection is theoretically low, however, that is not quite the end of the story. There is a great difference between theoretical effectiveness and real effectiveness, in practice, in the population as a whole. Theoretical effectiveness refers to ideal conditions, in which condoms are of good quality, are used correctly, and are used every time. These conditions rarely exist in practice. In Rakai, Uganda, for example, it was estimated that for the 4 percent of the population who used condoms consistently, the condoms provided only a 67 percent rate of effectiveness against

HIV infection.[13] In Finland, 37 percent of men and 34 percent of women who used condoms said condoms had failed. Among both men and women, one in every four said a condom had ruptured at some time.[14] Seventy-one percent of young people in the United States who had used a condom during the previous three months experienced at least one error problem: 41 percent forgot to use them, 31 percent experienced condom ruptures, and 15 percent had the condom slip off; only 16 percent were "consistent users."[15] These failures must be weighed against the real possibility of contracting a fatal infection.

Moreover, there is no evidence that inconsistent condom use provides *any* protection against HIV transmission.[16] On the contrary, there is a great deal of evidence suggesting that people who use condoms inconsistently may be at greater risk of infection than those who do not use them, probably because they tend to have a higher rate of other risk factors, such as multiple sexual partners and drug use.[17] Since so many condom users use them inconsistently, this problem must also be weighed against the possibility of contracting a fatal infection.

These are not concepts that can be communicated simply or quickly or even neutrally in a voluntary screening and personal counseling session.

Encouraging Voluntary Counseling and Testing

Voluntary counseling and testing (VCT) has been, and remains, a mainstay of the AIDS Establishment's approach to HIV prevention, largely because its value-neutrality is consistent with the AIDS Establishment's philosophical outlook. VCT campaigns tend to downplay underlying behaviors per se, and rely heavily on encouraging condom use. VCT was a favored intervention even before the recent and rapid increases in the availability of antiretroviral therapy, which has required a large increase in testing.

The assumption is that if people know their HIV status, they will adjust their behavior to protect themselves and others. U.N. Ambassador Richard Holbrook was merely expressing what had long been axiomatic when he wrote in the *Washington Post*,

> But isn't it obvious that AIDS will continue to spread more rapidly as long as 90 percent of those affected do not know their status? Wouldn't greater knowledge of one's status—held in the strictest confidence (an essential part of any testing program)—greatly modify behavior, both for those who are HIV-positive and for the large majority who, even in the worst-hit areas, are not infected? [18]

But testing alone does not directly influence incidence: *behavior* influences incidence. The question is, therefore, what is the impact of VCT on behavior and thus on HIV incidence?

The impact of VCT on behavior and on HIV incidence remains rather unimpressive. A recent randomized trial of VCT services in Zimbabwe concluded that even highly accessible VCT did not lead to declines in HIV incidence—and also that rapid testing appeared to have adverse behavioral consequences in some HIV-negative clients.[19] An earlier meta-analysis demonstrated that while in developing countries VCT may lead to some behavioral changes in those clients who are already HIV-positive, it does not seem to be effective as an instrument for primary prevention.[20]

A more recent study from Uganda likewise found that VCT neither changed behavior nor reduced HIV incidence. It suggested that HIV-negative people who accept repeated sessions of VCT constitute a special risk group because they persistently engage in risk-taking behavior.[21] A thorough 2005 review of the impact of VCT on risk-taking behavior and HIV incidence concluded that it would be difficult to assert that an increase in VCT would yield its hoped-for prevention benefits.[22]

VCT programs as currently devised seem to be insufficient as an HIV prevention strategy. This does not mean that counseling and testing are not important for other reasons or should be abandoned. It does mean that the substantial investment in VCT as a frontline of defense against HIV transmission is not based on the evidence and has not produced the anticipated results.

All VCT efforts should therefore be accompanied by rigorous risk avoidance campaigns, stressing mutual fidelity and abstinence, respect between the sexes, and healthy cultural norms of behavior. Finally, it is most instructive to recall also that HIV incidence and prevalence were declining in Uganda in the late 1980s and early 1990s, long before VCT services were even introduced by the Western donor community.

Treating Other Sexually Transmitted Infections

Another mainstay of the public health approach to AIDS prevention has been to treat *other* sexually transmitted infections (STIs) in order to reduce the transmission of HIV. Although the same behavior that accounts for an STI could also result in an HIV infection, this prevention strategy is not so much behavioral as it is biological. It is not meant to dissuade people from engaging in risky behavior in the first place. Treatment of the STI is specifically designed to provide a biological mechanism of protection for those exposed to the HIV virus by making it less likely to establish a foothold in the body.

The basis for the strategy rests on the assumption that some HIV infections can be attributed to another pre-existing untreated STI (by virtue of lesions, sores, and greater exposure of the virus to blood). In other words, all other things being equal, some HIV infections would not occur except for the presence of another STI. The World Health Organization has long asserted that the presence of an untreated STI increases the risk of both acquiring and transmitting HIV.[23] The related hypothesis—that better management and treatment of STIs would reduce HIV incidence more broadly in the general population—soon became conventional wisdom in the AIDS Establishment.

Initially, perhaps, this idea held some merit. One Tanzanian study found that the treatment of STIs yielded a reduction in HIV incidence close to 40 percent.[24]

However, five further randomized controlled trials were not able to demonstrate similar results.[25] In fact, these five other studies indicated that treatment of bacterial STIs had no effect on HIV.[26] These trials featured either the mass treatment of all members of the community for bacterial STIs or the treatment for bacterial STIs by means of syndromic management, that is, treating symptoms generally associated with bacterial STIs without necessarily identifying the specific pathogen responsible for morbidity. This approach is widely used for managing STIs in the developing world, where laboratory diagnostic facilities are uncommon; it is also more feasible in terms of costs and minimizes unwarranted delays in treatment.

Perhaps the initial success in Tanzania may have been attributable to the relatively early stage of the HIV epidemic; it remains open to speculation. Nonetheless, for all practical purposes, the results of every subsequent trial make the overwhelming body of evidence negative.

Although treatment of bacterial STIs has been ineffective in reducing HIV rates, most STIs in southern Africa are viral, suggesting the possibility that the treatment of viral infections might be more effective. However, despite some encouraging early indications, the evidence to date does not seem particularly promising. A 2007 article in the *New England Journal of Medicine*, for example, suggested that herpes simplex virus suppressive therapy may potentially help control HIV, but it remained unclear whether routine use of such therapy will provide benefit to patients by reducing the progression of HIV or benefit to the community by reducing transmission to others.[27] More conclusive evidence was published in the journal *Science* in 2008, showing that "two recent [randomized controlled trials] to prevent HIV acquisition by treating genital herpes have been similarly discouraging."[28]

Despite these highly relevant findings, this strategy of treating STIs has remained a fixture in HIV prevention among the AIDS Establishment. The World Health Organization now uses a bit more caution and says that "people with STIs *may* be at higher risk of acquiring or transmitting HIV infection," yet they assert that "programmes for the prevention and treatment of STIs, especially among populations at higher risk for sexual transmission of HIV, remain important elements of HIV prevention programmes."[29]

Treating STIs—which are a considerable source of morbidity in their own right—would be important even if there were no HIV epidemic, but it seems clear that we can expect minimal impact on HIV transmission from such a strategy, particularly in Africa's generalized epidemics.[30] Indeed, the AIDS Establishment's persistent reliance on this strategy as a major plank in efforts to curb HIV seems hard to justify.

Researchers at the University of Alberta in Edmonton, Canada, argued convincingly in an important article published in the *American Journal of Obstetrics and Gynecology* that in the face of discouraging results from "barrier methods" (condoms) and the treatment or "management" of infections, medical professionals, educators, and governments are confronted with two contrasting options: either accept high or rising rates of STIs as "inevitable or unavoidable" or focus on the actual, underlying behavior that leads to heightened susceptibility to infection.[31] Yet the latter is precisely what the World Health Organization resists at every turn. Its deep-seated reluctance to address in earnest the underlying sexual behavior seems to reveal a preference for an almost exclusively technical solution to the problem.

The technical way out of disease promises emancipation from whatever nature's verdict might otherwise be. It makes no pesky demands on behavior. On the contrary, in implicitly promising a lack of undesirable consequences, it subtly validates the activity itself: no harm, no foul. With sufficient technical advances, the prospect of disease or pregnancy could theoretically be eliminated, thus removing hindrances to the raw pursuit of sexual pleasure. Without technical measures, however, there would naturally be a greater incentive to cut back—to check sexual appetite—if only for pragmatic reasons. The promise of a technical solution to the AIDS epidemic, however remote, keeps unwelcome challenges to cherished notions of sexual liberation at bay.

Although their recommendation has gone unheeded by most of the AIDS Establishment, the Canadian researchers urged that prevention "initiatives focusing on primary prevention of behaviors predisposing individuals to [sexually transmitted disease] risk must be adopted," since "the promotion of optimal lifelong health can be achieved most effectively through delayed sexual debut, partner reduction, and the avoidance of risky sexual behaviors."[32]

This is sound, commonsense advice. When a person has more than one sex partner during the year, the risk of acquiring an STI such as chlamydia, gonorrhea, trichomoniasis, or human papillomavirus triples and is greater than the protective effect of condoms during those sexual relations.[33] A decrease in the number of sex partners has a greater impact on HIV transmission than the treatment of STIs or the use of condoms.[34] Even partial adoption of A and B can have a much more profound impact on the epidemic than treatment of STIs.

Ignoring Evidence

In many countries in sub-Saharan Africa, HIV transmission rates have remained high and even grown, despite a considerable increase in condom use. Condom sales in Botswana increased from one million in 1993 to three million in 2001, while HIV prevalence among pregnant urban women increased from 27 to 45 percent. In Cameroon, condom sales rose from six million to fifteen million in the same period, while HIV prevalence increased from 3 to 9 percent.[35]

There is great incongruence between the theoretical effectiveness of the condom at the individual level, and the public perception of its actual effectiveness at the population level. This crucial distinction is generally not well understood. This remains the case particularly in the Western media, even though respected researchers were pointing out as early as the year 2000 that "massive increases in condom use worldwide have not translated into demonstrably improved HIV control in the great majority of countries where they have occurred."[36]

An exhaustive review of the impact of condom promotion on actual HIV transmission in the developing world concluded that condoms have not been responsible for turning around any of the severe African epidemics. This rigorous study was originally commissioned by UNAIDS and conducted by researchers at the University of California at San Francisco. Dr. Norman Hearst, who led the study, was originally surprised by the results and found that they were not what "UNAIDS wanted to hear at all."[37]

Instead of welcoming the findings and adapting HIV prevention strategies accordingly, UNAIDS first tried to alter the findings and then refused to publish them. The findings were so threatening to UNAIDS that the researchers were finally forced to publish them on their own in another prestigious, though less visible, peer-reviewed journal, *Studies in Family Planning*.[38]

Meanwhile, explains Hearst, UNAIDS "released their own separate statement about how wonderful and effective condoms are. This did not have our names on it, nor would I have wanted it to."[39] Hearst had worked with the UNAIDS for years prior to this study but never received an explanation for their actions and soon sensed that he had been blacklisted.

This episode provides a disturbing glimpse into the priorities of the leading AIDS agency of the United Nations. Although normally quick to insist on the right to "accurate information" about condoms, in this case UNAIDS placed their own ideological preferences above the welfare of those whom they are charged with protecting. In fact, this flagrant disregard for highly relevant evidence reveals their relative lack of interest in questions of science; rather, they seem to "have considered the disease a profound threat to the ideology of the sexual revolution, and have at times put both the protection and the promotion of this ideology ahead of public health."[40] It would be difficult to avoid concluding that such actions fail others miserably, even by the standards of the most secular humanism.

While these findings proved a threat to UNAIDS, they prompted Hearst to remark, with great independence and integrity, that what is needed is to "move beyond debating how well condom promotion might work to examining how well it has."[41]

The evidence has led Hearst and other respected scientists to say that campaigns encouraging condom use will do more harm than good if they lead young people to have sexual relations, especially if the young people end up using condoms inconsistently and in situations where there is a high risk of transmission. A campaign promoting condom use does more harm than good if it fosters sexual practices that are riskier than those in which people would engage had they not been exposed to the campaign.

Riskier behaviors are associated with increases in HIV infection, and "this would seem to strengthen the argument that interventions are needed to lower the levels of higher-risk sexual activity," according to Harvard researcher Edward C. Green in his groundbreaking 2004 book, *Rethinking AIDS Prevention*. Green concludes that "adding condoms to high-risk behavior does not seem to have much impact on the consequences of the behavior. Condoms evidently do not protect against HIV infection as well as they are supposed to."[42]

Promotion of condoms, voluntary testing and counseling, and treatment of sexually transmitted infections have had a negligible impact on HIV incidence in Africa. Nevertheless, these risk reduction interventions still form the backbone of the World Health Organization's "comprehensive" HIV prevention strategy. This alone would seem to raise serious questions. Indeed, the World Health Organization was criticized in 2007 more broadly—regarding a host of other health matters—for rarely using systematic reviews or concise summaries of findings in developing their recommendations.[43]

Although the contributions that risk avoidance behaviors have made in national success stories have been decisive, and risk reduction measures a major disappointment, there are certainly instances where a risk reduction strategy has helped avert infection. Condoms, for example, may have protected some individuals some of the time. But they have not had a protective epidemiological impact at the population level. Therefore, from a purely pragmatic point of view, there remain large and serious concerns about the practical impact and efficacy of risk reduction strategies. Pointing this out is one thing; pointing out that some people are uneasy about the messages that the strategies convey—about their underlying moral and philosophical foundations—is another.

Notes

1. D. Wilson, "Partner Reduction and the Prevention of HIV/AIDS," *British Medical Journal* 328.7444 (April 10, 2004): 848–849.

2. Daniel Low-Beer, "Global Failures and Local Successes in HIV Prevention," online letter to the editor, *British Medical Journal*, July 9, 2003, http://www.bmj.com/cgi/eletters/326/7403/1389#34209.

3. U.N. General Assembly, Twenty-sixth Special Session, *Declaration of Commitment on HIV/AIDS*, August 2, 2001 (A/RES/S-26/2), para. 52, http://www.un.org/ga/aids/docs/aress262.pdf.

4. Joint U.N. Program on HIV/AIDS and World Health Organization, *AIDS Epidemic Update: December 2005* (UNAIDS/05.19E), http://www.unaids.org/epi/2005/doc/EPIupdate2005_pdf_en/epiupdate2005_en.pdf.

5. Ibid., 25.

6. World AIDS Campaign, *Stop AIDS—Keep the Promise: 2005 and Beyond*, 2005, 8–9, http://data.unaids.org/WAC/wac05_overview_en.pdf.

7. UN *Declaration of Commitment*, 2001, emphasis added.

8. Peter Piot, "Global Health: America's Response," interview by David Brancaccio, *NOW* documentary, PBS, November 4, 2005, http://www.pbs.org/now/transcript/transcript NOWGL_full.html.

9. Michael Czerny, "The Pope and AIDS in Africa: A Human and Spiritual Wake Up Call," *Thinking Faith* (March 25, 2009), http://www.thinkingfaith.org/articles/200903251.htm.

10. Wilson, "Partner Reduction."

11. Susan C. Weller and Karen R. Davis, "Condom Effectiveness in Reducing Heterosexual HIV Transmission," *Cochrane Database of Systematic Reviews* issue 3, article CD003255, 2001.

12. Ibid.

13. Ahmed et al., "HIV Incidence and Sexually Transmitted Disease Prevalence Associated with Condom Use: A Population Study in Rakai, Uganda," *AIDS* 15.16 (November 9, 2009): 2171–2179.

14. Anna-Leena Kirkkola, Kari Mattila, and Irma Virjo, "Problems with Condoms: A Population-Based Study among Finnish Men and Women," *European Journal of Contraception and Reproductive Health Care* 10.2 (June 2005): 87–92.

15. Gabriela Paz-Bailey et al., "The Effect of Correct and Consistent Condom Use on Chlamydial and Gonococcal Infection among Urban Adolescents," *Archives of Pediatrics and Adolescent Medicine* 159.6 (2005): 536–542.

16. Ahmed et al., "HIV Incidence and Sexually Transmitted Disease Prevalence."

17. Norman Hearst and Sanny Chen, "Condom Promotion for AIDS Prevention in the Developing World: Is It Working?" *Studies in Family Planning* 35.1 (March 2004): 39–47.

18. Richard Holbrook, "Sorry, But AIDS Testing Is Critical," *Washington Post*, January 4, 2006.

19. Elizabeth L. Corbett et al., "HIV Incidence During a Cluster-Randomized Trial of Two Strategies Providing Voluntary Counselling and Testing at the Workplace, Zimbabwe," *AIDS* 21.4 (February 19, 2007): 483–489.

20. Lance S. Weinhardt et al., "Effects of HIV Counseling and Testing on Sexual Risk Behavior: A Meta-Analytic Review of Published Research, 1985–1997," *American Journal of Public Health* 89.9 (1999): 1397–1405.

21. Joseph K. B. Matovu et al., "Repeat Voluntary HIV Counseling and Testing, Sexual Risk Behavior and HIV Incidence in Rakai, Uganda," *AIDS and Behavior* 11.1 (January 2007): 71–78.

22. Peter Glick, *Scaling up HIV Voluntary Counseling and Testing in Africa: What Can Evaluation Studies Tell Us about Potential Prevention Impacts?* SAGA Working Paper (Ithaca, NY: Strategies and Analysis for Growth and Access, March 2005), http://pdf.dec.org/pdf_docs/PNADC113.pdf.

23. World Health Organization, *Global Prevalence and Incidence of Selected Curable Sexually Transmitted Infections: Overview and Estimates* (Geneva: WHO, 2001), http://www.who.int/hiv/pub/sti/who_hiv_aids_2001.02.pdf.

24. Malcolm Potts et al., "Reassessing HIV Prevention," *Science* 320.5877 (May 9, 2008): 749–750.

25. Matthew Hanley, "A Realistic Strategy for Fighting African AIDS," *MercatorNet*, February 28, 2008, http://www.mercatornet.com/articles/a_realistic_strategy_for_fighting_african_aids.

26. Potts et al., "Reassessing HIV Prevention."

27. Lawrence Corey, "Synergistic Copathogens: HIV-1 and HSV-2," *New England Journal of Medicine* 356.8 (February 22, 2007): 854–856.

28. Potts et al., "Reassessing HIV Prevention."

29. World Health Organization, *Priority Interventions: HIV/AIDS Prevention, Treatment and Care in the Health Sector,* version 1.2, Geneva, 2009, 15, emphasis added, http://www.who.int/hiv/pub/priority_interventions_web.pdf.

30. Hanley, "Realistic Strategy"; P. Sangani, G. Rutherford, and G. E. Kennedy, "Population-Based Interventions for Reducing Sexually Transmitted Infections, Including HIV Infection," *Cochrane Database of Systematic Reviews* 3, article CD001220, 2004.

31. Stephen J. Genuis and Shelagh K. Genuis, "Managing the Sexually Transmitted Disease Pandemic: A Time for Reevaluation," *American Journal of Obstetrics and Gynecology* 191.4 (October 2004): 1103–1112.

32. Ibid.

33. Ineke G. Stolte, John B. F. de Wit, Marion Kolader et al., "Association between 'Safer Sex Fatigue' and Rectal Gonorrhea Is Mediated by Unsafe Sex with Casual Partners among HIV-Positive Homosexual Men," *Sexually Transmitted Diseases* 33.4 (April 2006): 201–208; N. V. Revzina and R. J. DiClemente, "Prevalence and Incidence of Human Papillomavirus Infection in Women in the USA: A Systematic Review," *International Journal of STD and AIDS* 16.8 (2005): 528–537; Salvatore Vaccarella et al., "Sexual Behavior, Condom Use, and Human Papillomavirus: Pooled Analysis of the IARC Human Papillomavirus Prevalence Surveys," *Cancer Epidemiology, Biomarkers and Prevention* 15.2 (February 2006): 326–333; and Ralph J. DiClemente et al., "Reducing Risk Exposures to Zero and Not Having Multiple Partners: Findings That

Inform Evidence-Based Practices Designed to Prevent STD Acquisition," *International Journal of STD and AIDS* 16.12 (December 2005): 816–818.

34. Edward C. Green, testimony before U.S. Senate Committee on Foreign Relations, May 19, 2003, *Fighting AIDS in Uganda: What Went Right?* 108th Cong., 1st sess., http://foreign.senate .gov/hearings/2003/hrg030519p.html.

35. Hearst and Chen, "Condom Promotion."

36. John Richens, John Imrie, and Andrew Copas, "Condoms and Seat Belts: The Parallels and the Lessons," *Lancet* 355.9201 (January 29, 2000): 400–403.

37. Curtis Abraham, "UNAIDS and Myth of Condoms' Efficacy against AIDS," *East African*, February 7, 2009, http://www.the eastafrican.co.ke/news/-/2558/525956/-/rku48lz/-/index.html.

38. Hearst and Chen, "Condom Promotion."

39. Abraham, "UNAIDS and Myth."

40. Douglas A. Sylva, "AIDS and the Ideological Barrier: The Threat to Sexual Liberation," *Ethics & Medics* 33.12 (December 2008): 4.

41. Sue Ellin Browder, "Why Condoms Will Never Stop AIDS in Africa," *Inside Catholic,* May 31, 2006, http://insidecatholic .com/Joomla/index.php?option=com_content&task=view& id=182&Itemid=12.

42. Edward C. Green, *Rethinking AIDS Prevention: Learning from Successes in Developing Countries* (Westport, CT: Praeger, 2003), 111.

43. A. D. Oxman, J. N. Lavis, and A. Fretheim, "Use of Evidence in WHO Recommendations," *World Hospitals and Health Services* 43.2 (2007):14–20, reprinted from *Lancet* 369.9576 (June 2, 2007): 1883–1889.

V

Confronting the Data

Evidence for the influence of other factors on HIV transmission needs to be assessed with care. Among these factors are poverty, the practice of having multiple or intergenerational sexual partners, and the phenomenon of risk compensation, which are considered here.

HIV/AIDS and Poverty

The AIDS Establishment has frequently asserted that poverty—not just material deprivation but food or economic insecurity and exploitive inequality—causes AIDS, and therefore that improving material conditions will lead to a decrease in AIDS.[1] This argument, though worthy of serious evaluation, has also tended to divert attention from the actual source of HIV transmission, which is behavior.

It is true that in some cases poverty can be a decisive factor contributing to the behaviors that lead to HIV transmission. External factors (whether economic or cultural) would increase HIV transmission inasmuch as they result in exploitation and exposure to HIV through multiple sexual partners. For example, poor women may become involved in "transactional sex" or the commercial sex trade in an effort to get out of poverty, placing both themselves and their sex partners at greater risk. It would be wrong to conclude, however, that HIV transmission is mainly a consequence of economic status; indeed, many studies have revealed nearly the opposite.[2]

Unlike tuberculosis or cholera, "AIDS is not necessarily a disease of poverty, but AIDS deepens and prolongs poverty."[3] In fact, higher income and education levels are associated with higher-risk behaviors and increased HIV infection.[4] In *Rethinking AIDS Prevention*, Edward Green refers to three Cs as risk factors: "cash, car and cell phone."[5] People with these assets typically are able to attract more sexual partners—and thereby end up furthering HIV transmission.

The wealthier African countries (South Africa, Botswana, Swaziland, and even Zimbabwe prior to its recent collapse) have the continent's highest HIV infection rates (between 25 and 40 percent of the population is infected), while some of the poorer countries (Somalia, Guinea, Liberia, Mali, and Eritrea) have the lowest. In Zambia, HIV prevalence notably increases with the level of education, ranging from 13 percent in women with less than primary education to 26 percent among those with college or university education.[6] One study carried out in Tanzania found a strong, positive association between greater household wealth and HIV prevalence, perhaps because wealthier men and women have more means for having multiple and concurrent sex partners (Figure 6, *next page*).

An analysis of the 2003–2005 Demographic and Health Surveys, which are funded by the United States, reveals that "contrary to evidence for other infectious diseases and theoretical expectations, in sub-Saharan Africa HIV prevalence is not disproportionately higher among adults living in poorer households."[7] Policy makers, therefore, need to adjust to the reality that HIV prevalence is not necessarily higher among the poorer.[8]

In fact, while AIDS is not primarily or exclusively a disease of the poor, acquiring HIV/AIDS clearly prolongs and exacerbates poverty and can be considered a principal source of poverty.[9] HIV/AIDS itself "generates new poverty," reducing income as well as depreciating human, physical, natural, and social assets.[10] UNAIDS data show that household income in Africa can fall by 30 to 60 percent as a result of HIV/AIDS. At the same time household spending on health care can quadruple, while spending on food can decrease substantially (by as much as 41 percent).[11]

HIV/AIDS is thus unlike many other diseases in that greater material assets do not protect against infection, because HIV transmission is ultimately behavioral in nature and is influenced by cultural norms relating to sexuality. Peter Glick of Cornell University, after reviewing the variables involved, concluded that there is considerable evidence to refute the "popular view that

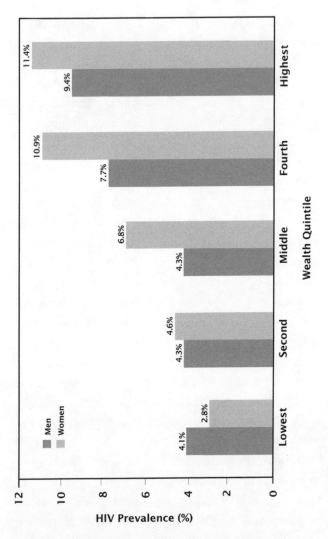

Figure 6. HIV prevalence by wealth quintile. These 2003–2004 data from Tanzania show an increased HIV prevalence with greater wealth. Similar findings have been reported for

the best way to reduce AIDS is to reduce poverty."[12] The Ethiopian Catholic Church echoed this perception by saying, "Since wealth, education, information, or youth, in and of themselves, do not guarantee protection against this virus, it further points to the urgent need to form consciences, creatively articulate and promote human and spiritual values, and reinforce norms of behavior that respect man's capacity to love."[13]

Addressing very real needs for greater human development, alleviation of poverty, and respect between the sexes does not conflict with promoting abstinence and fidelity. Conversely, A and B facilitate the practical pursuit of those social goods, will ultimately lead to reduced HIV transmission, and can only help contribute to economic improvement.

One final note: Very poor women who resort to prostitution to survive or to feed their children do not wish to be in that situation. They need alternative sources of

---

other sub-Saharan countries. The fact that AIDS, unlike tuberculosis or cholera, is not primarily a disease of the poor strikes many as surprising, but as Shelton et al. note that "the difference in prevalence for women between the lowest and highest wealth quintile is four-fold." SOURCE: From James D. Shelton, Michael M. Cassell, and Jacob Adetunji, "Is Poverty or Wealth at the Root of HIV?" *Lancet* 366.9491 (September 24, 2005), 1058, based on data from the Tanzania Commission for AIDS, National Bureau of Statistics, and ORC Macro, Tanzania HIV/AIDS Indicator Survey 2003–2004 (Calverton, MD: TACAIDS, NBS, and ORC, 2005), 75.

income, which can be provided through training and income-generating projects. Merely settling for risk reduction sends a message that they and their children do not matter and can continue to be used and abused.

Multiple Sexual Partners

In parts of southern Africa, the current infection rate among women between ages fifteen and nineteen is three to four times that of their male counterparts. In South Africa, young females with sex partners more than five years older have much higher rates of infection than those who do not have older partners.[14] This indicates a particular vulnerability for young women and the dangers of cross-generational sex. For these reasons some voices within the AIDS Establishment are striving to redefine the AIDS prevention paradigm, following the mantra of "lead with partner reduction and focus on adult men."[15] This is a significant development, since the unquestioned mantra had always been "lead with C."

In 2006, an international group of HIV prevention technical experts convened in Lesotho in 2006 to review and discuss trends related to HIV transmission in southern Africa. They recommended that an essential priority of international HIV prevention guidelines should be to "address gender issues especially from the perspective of *male involvement and responsibility* ... specifically to reduce multiple and concurrent partnerships, intergenerational/age-disparate sex, and sexual violence."[16]

At the same time, however, as David Wilson of the World Bank and Daniel Halperin of the Harvard School of Public Health pointed out in the *Lancet*, "it is striking that a comparison of gender equality and HIV prevalence across African countries shows a strong positive, not negative, association."[17] In Botswana, for example, where the epidemic is severe, men and women enjoy relative equality. The much poorer Niger, with much more inequality between men and women, has very low HIV prevalence (0.7 percent). This would suggest that gender inequality per se is not the driving force behind HIV transmission, but rather the extent of multiple partnerships (as well as differing male circumcision patterns mentioned earlier).

In 2006, James Shelton of USAID wrote an article in the *Lancet* refuting commonly held myths about generalized HIV epidemics. In discussing the issue of gender equity and HIV/AIDS, he observed that the role of male behavior, though more widely recognized, cannot be held entirely accountable. He noted that women who have multiple partners are also a significant contributor to the severity of generalized epidemics.[18]

Thus we cannot adequately confront HIV transmission without addressing, more specifically, the issue of multiple sexual partners. Honest reflection about the cause (proximate determinants) of HIV transmission is possible; indeed, it is the essential first step in formulating just responses. This means that the value-based dimensions of having multiple sexual partners and, by extension, other harmful cultural attitudes or practices must be reexamined.

The national AIDS commissions for Kenya, Tanzania, and Uganda have asserted that "the centrality of culture must be addressed more rigorously."[19] For example, the cultural practice of wife inheritance heightens vulnerability to HIV transmission in some parts of Kenya. When a husband dies, tradition indicates that his widow is to be taken in by a brother or another male relative. This practice once served to protect and provide for the widow, but this central dimension of the practice is now often neglected. The mandate for the widow to have sexual relations, however, has been retained. In fact, the practice has by and large devolved into a sexual ritual to be performed—even if not by the traditionally prescribed person. Sometimes anyone will have to do. Driving through rural west Kenya, we once picked up a man who identified himself as a "wife inheritor"; he made himself available to perform the "cleansing" that some imagined was necessary.

Malawi has also taken a step in this direction, stating in its national AIDS strategy that "culture is one of the underlying determining factors in the course of the epidemic," and it has identified a series of harmful cultural practices that must be addressed. As in Kenya, there is widow and widower inheritance in Malawi. In addition, they identified other practices, such as forced sex for young girls coming of age, consensual adultery for childless couples, wife- and husband-exchange, and temporary husband replacement.[20] Other risky practices include the use of unsterilized skin piercing and cutting instruments for scarification, circumcision, ear piercing, and tattooing. Modifying these traditional customs so that they are still able to achieve their cultural purpose without exposing people to HIV infection takes on special urgency.

This process of exploring and modifying harmful cultural attitudes and practices is promising, albeit not without tension. After all, there is an inherent and underlying incongruence between the cultural acceptance of the multiple sexual partnerships, on the one hand, and the simultaneous belief that HIV infection results from having engaged in "illicit" behavior. Why, for example, would there be a debilitating sense of stigma in contracting HIV if people are truly expected to have multiple sex partners (as is commonly said)?

In the final analysis, respect for the dignity and value all persons, the just treatment of women, and the responsibilities that come with sexuality must be promoted. Dignity and justice, though underemphasized, are highly relevant concepts for HIV prevention, and are surely pertinent to the overall response to the AIDS epidemic.

Dignity is commonly and properly invoked in terms of providing compassionate care to people living with HIV/ AIDS, especially in desperate circumstances in which palliative care is limited. Yet dignity is just as relevant to prevention for young or otherwise vulnerable people who are not infected. Taking the dignity of every person seriously means fully respecting their inherent worth as persons, not consigning them to circumstances of inescapable peril, degradation, or exploitation and striving merely to make it all "safer." It means settling for nothing less than their integral well-being. Risk reduction measures abandon the concept of integral well-being and propose a one-dimensional "solution." This often shortchanges the full measure of dignity due to each person; it treats people as objects to be managed rather than participants in their own authentic development.

Justice is often invoked in terms of ensuring that African countries have the same access to medication as developed countries. Yet justice certainly applies to the realm of interpersonal relationships as well. The exploitation and misuse of others (like commercial sex workers or multiple sexual partners) is an injustice, whether or not HIV is part of the picture. It may be disconcerting to admit this; it hits closer to home and threatens the West's cherished sexual libertinism. It also reeks of judgmentalism, which is the ultimate violation of political correctness, even among those who are otherwise inclined to fight for justice. It is more fashionable to identify wider structural issues like the economy (poverty) or access to medicines as the important AIDS-related justice issues. We should continue to address those issues, but we also need to recognize that interpersonal injustice is inextricably intertwined with the AIDS epidemic as well as with many other contemporary social ills. This painful truth could be better factored into anti-AIDS campaigns.

One HIV-positive young woman whom we met at Nsambya Hospital in Kampala, Uganda, told us how crushed she was by the circumstances that led to her contracting AIDS. She had been a happy girl, poor but well adjusted to her surroundings. Her parents died young, and an older man offered to pay her school fees. Soon he asked for her to come live with him. Her caretaker, an older sister, agreed. It was not long before she contracted HIV; she became pregnant and her baby died from AIDS. Her unforgettable message to us amounted to an impassioned plea for justice, for safeguarding human dignity: "Tell the parents and the adults out there to look out for their children—otherwise none of this would have happened." What pained her so sharply was that no one stood up for her when she was young and vulnerable. No one recognized her dignity; no one insisted she be treated justly. Had there been adults in her life to protect her, she could have been spared the trauma of exploitation.

To imagine that the destructive effects of multiple concurrent partnerships—not to mention the injustices of rape, coercion, poverty, and abuse—including the heightened risk of spreading HIV, are to be satisfactorily and effectively addressed by mere recourse to condoms or other risk reduction measures is not only folly but fatalistic. Achieving dignity and justice means paying attention to the practical indignities and injustices that foster HIV transmission. One aspect of social transformation is profound respect for the particular and essential dignity of women and young people and for the justice due them. Dignity and justice are effectively pursued through abstinence and fidelity.

Risk Compensation

A further weakness in the risk reduction approach is now receiving more attention in scientific circles: people may increase risk-taking behavior because they perceive themselves to be at less risk due to a technological innovation. This behavioral disinhibition is sometimes called "risk compensation" because the benefits of an intervention designed to reduce risk can be offset if enough people who use it become careless about preventive behaviors or give them up.[21] For example, people who made greater use of sunscreen suffered an increase in skin cancer because they compensated for the sunscreen's protective effects with longer exposures to the sun.[22]

John Richens, a British scientist who has done pioneering research on this phenomenon, argued in a landmark 2000 *Lancet* article that risk compensation was responsible for the initial failure of seatbelt laws to prevent deaths in traffic accidents. Many drivers assumed the seatbelt would protect them even if they drove more recklessly or under the effects of alcohol.[23] In the same article Richens drew the parallel to condoms and sexually transmitted infections like AIDS by noting, "A vigorous condom-promotion policy could increase rather than decrease unprotected sexual exposure, if it has the unintended effect of encouraging greater sexual activity."[24]

Risk compensation has been observed with a number of HIV/AIDS-preventive measures, such as the promotion of condom use, the introduction of antiretroviral therapy, and post-exposure prophylaxis (taking antiretroviral therapy soon after suspected exposure to the virus in hopes that the virus will not take hold in the body).[25] Other measures like voluntary counseling and testing and the treatment of sexually transmitted infections may also have a disinhibiting effect.[26] If A and B were properly emphasized as the safest and most effective way of preventing HIV infection, with the warning that condoms substantially reduce the risk but do not eliminate it, those who choose condom use would be better informed about the concept of risk reduction and might be more motivated to avoid the slippery slope of risk compensation.[27]

Risk compensation surfaced as a major theme during Pope Benedict XVI's trip to Cameroon in March 2009. A reporter asked the Pope to defend the Church's promotion of monogamy and opposition to condoms in the fight against AIDS, especially since such positions are "frequently considered unrealistic and ineffective." He responded in part by saying that "the scourge cannot be resolved by distributing condoms; quite the contrary, we risk worsening the problem." This prompted a fresh, if predictable, round of scorn from the Western press. France went so far as to say his statements represent a threat to public health. The *New York Times*—echoing the standard view of the AIDS Establishment—claimed, just hours after the Pope's remarks, that he "deserves no credence when he distorts scientific findings about the value of condoms in slowing the spread of the AIDS virus."[28]

Edward C. Green debunks that conventional wisdom, writing, "I am a liberal on social issues and it's difficult to admit, but the Pope is indeed right. The best evidence we have shows that condoms do not work as an intervention intended to reduce HIV infection rates in Africa."[29] Green concludes that what "we see in fact is an association between greater condom use and higher infection rates."

We have many empirically documented examples of this phenomenon. In Uganda, for example, a state-of-the-art condom promotion program found that the intervention group of eighteen- to thirty-year-olds used more condoms but also reported having significantly more partners than the control group. In the final analysis, the intervention group was at higher risk than the control group, even though the former had higher condom use.[30] These findings have been cited elsewhere in the scientific literature to demonstrate that behavioral disinhibition "is real."[31] It has also been argued that the promotion of condoms at an early stage proved counterproductive in Botswana, whereas the lack of condom promotion during the 1980s and early 1990s contributed to the relative success of strategies to change behavior in Uganda.[32]

These findings should prompt serious reconsideration of the dominant approach to HIV prevention advocated by the AIDS Establishment. They call into question how well these interventions have lived up to one of the most cherished principles and the first maxim in medicine and public health, "do no harm" (*primum non nocere*). This awareness also helps explain the AIDS Establishment's reluctance to acknowledge the decisive contributions of abstinence and fidelity and to give them the emphasis they deserve. This raises further interesting questions: Might there be something flawed in the philosophical and cultural assumptions on which these interventions are based? Ideas, after all, have consequences.

John Richens notes that demonstrating or precisely quantifying disinhibition in matters of sexual health is very difficult.[33] But he has pleaded for a "stronger focus on interventions that can be shown to truly reshape individual's willingness to expose themselves to the risks of HIV."[34] He has also pointed out that efforts to restrain behavior would confront entrenched forces within the culture, such as the "present climate of sexual freedom and the media portrayal of sex ... It would raise suspicions that whoever was delivering the message was acting from a moral standpoint."[35]

He has worried that scientific work in this area of risk compensation may be "misused" by religious or family-oriented groups, but has also admitted that the concept remains "off-limits" in the public health community, as it is perceived as a threat by those with vested professional interests. There are condoms to be sold, new markets to be opened, grants to be awarded, prestigious articles to be published. The concept thus threatens many livelihoods as well as cherished values of modern Western culture,

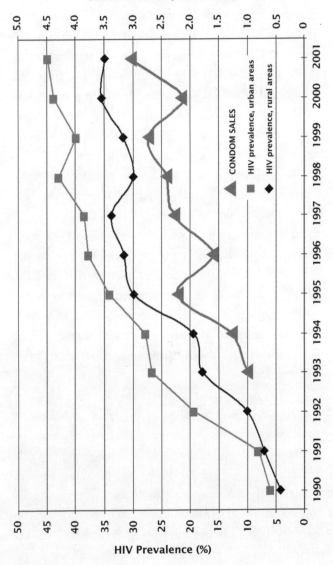

Condom Sales (in millions)

HIV Prevalence (%)

CONDOM SALES
HIV prevalence, urban areas
HIV prevalence, rural areas

which prizes complete sexual autonomy and expects that such autonomy should be without consequences and free from judgment. Failing to champion these cultural values or appearing to oppose them—even if only by presenting evidence which punctures the narrative of risk reduction's supreme effectiveness—can derail a career.

Internal data from the nongovernmental organization PSI (Population Services International), which is the largest American distributor of condoms around the world, also indicate that rising condom sales over time have coincided with rising HIV prevalence in African countries like Botswana and Cameroon, precisely where the Pope visited (Figure 7). These findings have been presented at professional venues and circulated in professional correspondence but not widely publicized. For those with a market to protect, the knowledge that their product may actually be contributing to the problem needs to be carefully managed.

FIGURE 7. HIV prevalence and condom sales. This graph shows the rise in HIV prevalence among pregnant women in Botswana from 1990 to 2001 even as condom sales increased. As indicated earlier (p. 71), condom sales rose in Cameroon from six million to fifteen million between 1993 and 2001, while HIV prevalence increased from 3 to 9 percent. These trends do not prove causation, but they do suggest a lack of epidemiological impact. SOURCE: Edward C. Green, "A Summary of ABC Evidence," presentation to the Presidential Advisory Council on HIV/AIDS, March 29, 2004, slide 13, based on data provided by PSI (Population Services International.

This organization, Population Services International, aware of these trends, has not faced harsh criticism of the kind routinely aimed at Pope Benedict by the Western press. On the contrary, it remains an ensconced fixture in the AIDS Establishment, where they find shelter with fellow travelers under the mantle of "objectivity." Thus, while many errors about AIDS prevention are committed in good faith and with humanitarian intentions, and while some discrepancies among scientists are due to diverging and sometimes difficult interpretations of empirical data, commercial interests certainly also play a role.

Many Africans perceive this. The Congolese theologian Benezet Bujo, for example, writes that "for the countries of the Third World ... we wonder if in the end, the manufacturers and merchants of condoms are not obsessed by money alone, as is the case for the sale of arms where human life no longer plays any role."[36] Bujo has a number of other pertinent observations to make on the subject.

"According to African wisdom," he writes, "a disease is always an indication that something in human relations is wrong."[37] Condom promotion simply cannot address this kind of breakdown in human relations. It cannot heal that discord or patch it over. It instead encourages "the consumer mentality of the modern world" and "reduces sex to the level of consumer goods."[38] This only perpetuates conflict and pain in human relations instead of offering the prospect of authentic healing or fulfillment. It also strips away many traditional African cultural understandings with respect to sex, discipline, responsibility, family and community. In essence, the "indiscriminate distribution of condoms ultimately wipes out African culture."[39]

He insists that if the West were truly interested in helping Africa, they "should offer their support in such a way that the African people can recover their spiritual and moral immunity, which cannot be underestimated even if it does not offer or replace a technical solution for AIDS."[40]

Notes

1. Peter Glick, *Reproductive Health and Behavior, HIV/AIDS, and Poverty in Africa*, SAGA Working Paper (Ithaca, NY: Strategies and Analysis for Growth and Access, May 2007), http://www.saga.cornell.edu/images/wp219.pdf. Glick largely refutes this theory in his paper.

2. James D. Shelton, Michael M. Cassell, and Jacob Adetunji, "Is Poverty or Wealth at the Root of HIV?" *Lancet* 366.9491 (September 24–30, 2005): 1057–1058.

3. Peter Piot, keynote address, in U.N. Administrative Committee on Coordination, Sub-Committee on Nutrition, *Nutrition and HIV/AIDS*, Report of the Twenty-eighth Session Symposium, Nairobi, Kenya, April 3–4, 2001, Nutrition Policy Paper 20 (Geneva: UN ACC/SCN, 2001).

4. Edward C. Green, *Rethinking AIDS Prevention: Learning from Successes in Developing Countries* (Westport, CT: Praeger, 2003), 313.

5. Ibid.

6. Edward C. Green, "Poverty Does Not Mean That Effective AIDS Prevention Is Impossible," *Share the World's Resources*, January 29, 2006, http://www.stwr.org/health-education

-shelter/poverty-does-not-mean-that-effective-aids-prevention
-is-impossible.html.

7. Vinod Mishra et al., *A Study of the Association of HIV Infection with Wealth in Sub-Saharan Africa*, DHS working paper 31, Macro International for USAID, January 2007, iii, http://www.measuredhs.com/pubs/pdf/WP31/WP31. See also Vinod Mishra et al., "HIV Infection Does Not Disproportionately Affect the Poorer in Sub-Saharan Africa," *AIDS* 21, suppl. 7 (November 2007): s17–s28.

8. Mishra et al., *Study of the Association of HIV Infection*.

9. Roger Thurow, "AIDS Fuels Famine in Africa," *Wall Street Journal*, July 9, 2003; and U.N. Administrative Committee on Coordination, Sub-Committee on Nutrition, *Nutrition and HIV/AIDS*, Report of the Twenty-eighth Session Symposium, Nairobi, Kenya, April 3–4, 2001, Nutrition Policy Paper 20 (Geneva: UN ACC/SCN, 2001).

10. Winford Masanjala, "The Poverty-HIV/AIDS Nexus in Africa: A Livelihood Approach," *Social Science and Medicine* 64.5 (March 2007): 1032–1041.

11. J. Parker, I. Singh and K. Hattel, *The Role of Microfinance in the Fight against HIV/AIDS—A Report to UNAIDS* (Bethesda, MD: Development Alternatives, September 15, 2000), http://www.microfinancegateway.org/gm/document-1.9.29154/2737_file_02737.pdf.

12. Peter Glick, *Reproductive Health and Behavior*.

13. Ethiopian Catholic Bishops, "Love As Our Main Tool of Overcoming HIV/AIDS," pastoral letter, Addis Ababa, February 25, 2007, 31.

14. David Stanton, "Evidence vs. Conventional Wisdom: AIDS Prevention in the Twenty-first Century," presented at the Johns Hopkins University, Baltimore, Maryland, March 13, 2006,

slide 29, based on data from O. Shisana et al., *South African National HIV Prevalence, HIV Incidence, Behaviour and Communication Survey* (Cape Town, South Africa: HSRC Press, 2005), 61, http://www.hsrcpress.ac.za/product.php?product id=2134.

15. Stanton, "Evidence vs. Conventional Wisdom," slide 43.

16. See Southern African Development Community, *Expert Think Tank Meeting on HIV Prevention in High-Prevalence Countries in Southern Africa: Report,* Maseru, Lesotho, May 10–12, 2006 (Gaborone, Botswana: SADC, 2006), 8, original emphasis.

17. David Wilson and Daniel T. Halperin, "'Know Your Epidemic, Know Your Response': A Useful Approach If We Get It Right," *Lancet* 372.9637 (August 9, 2008): 424.

18. James Shelton, "Ten Myths and One Truth about Generalized HIV Epidemics," *Lancet* 370.9602 (December 1, 2007): 1809.

19. Women of Uganda Network, "The Arusha Commitments of Gender and HIV/AIDS: From Policy to Practice in East Africa," draft, 2003, http://www.wougnet.org/Documents/ UNIFEM/arusha_genderhiv.html.

20. International Labour Organization, *Malawi National HIV/ AIDS Policy,* final draft, June 2003, 24, http://www.ilo.org/ public/english/protection/trav/aids/laws/malawi1.pdf; and FASU Consultancy and Maternal Life International, *AIDS Cultural Change Programme 2001–2006: Operation Phase 2004–2006* (Lilongwe, Malawi, and Butte, MT: FAMLI, 2006), 17.

21. Michael M. Cassell et al., "Risk Compensation: The Achilles' Heel of Innovations in HIV Prevention?" *British Medical Journal* 332.7541 (March 11, 2006): 605–607.

22. Philippe Autier et al., "Sunscreen Use, Wearing Clothes, and Number of Nevi in 6- to 7-Year-Old European Children. European Organization for Research and Treatment of Cancer Melanoma Cooperative Group," *Journal of the National Cancer Institute* 90.24 (December 16, 1998): 1873–1880.

23. John Richens, John Imrie, and Andrew Copas, "Condoms and Seat Belts: The Parallels and the Lessons," *Lancet* 355.9201 (January 29, 2000): 400–403

24. Ibid., 401.

25. David Wilson and Joy de Beyer, "Male Circumcision: Evidence and Implications," *World Bank HIV/AIDS Monitoring and Evaluation: Getting Results.* World Bank Global HIV/AIDS Program, March 2006.

26. John Richens, John Imrie, and Helen Weiss, "HIV Risk: Is It Possible to Dissuade People from Having Unsafe Sex?" *Journal of the Royal Statistical Society: Series A (Statistics in Society)* 166.2 (June 2003): 207–221.

27. Jokin de Irala and Alvaro Alonso, "Changes in Sexual Behaviors to Prevent HIV: The Need for Comprehensive Information," *Lancet* 368.9549 (November 18, 2006): 1749–1750.

28. "The Pope on Condoms and AIDS," *New York Times*, March 17, 2009. http://www.nytimes.com/2009/03/18/opinion/18wed2 .html.

29. Edward C. Green, interview with *Ilsussidiario*, March 23, 2009, http://www.ilsussidiario.net/articolo.aspx?articolo=14614. See also Edward C. Green, "The Pope May Be Right," *Washington Post*, March 29, 2009, http://www.washingtonpost. com/wp-dyn/content/article/2009/03/27/AR2009032702825 _pf.html.

30. Phoebe Kajubi et al., "Increasing Condom Use without Reducing HIV Risk: Results of a Controlled Community Trial in

Uganda," *Journal of Acquired Immune Deficiency Syndromes* 40.1 (September 1, 2005): 77–82.

31. James D. Shelton, "Confessions of a Condom Lover," *Lancet* 368.9551 (December 2, 2006): 1947.

32. Tim Allen and Suzette Heald, "HIV/AIDS Policy in Africa: What Has Worked in Uganda and What Has Failed in Botswana?" *Journal of International Development* 16.8 (November 8, 2004): 1141–1154.

33. The authors are indebted here to personal correspondence with Richens.

34. Richens, Imrie, and Weiss, "HIV Risk."

35. Ibid.

36. Benezet Bujo, "What Morality for the Problem of AIDS in Africa?" in *AIDS and the Church in Africa: To Shepherd the Church Family of God in Africa in the Age of AIDS,* ed. Michael Czerny for the African Jesuit AIDS Network (Nairobi: Pauline Publications, 2005), 57.

37. Raymond Downing, "African Perspective on AIDS Crisis Differs from West," *National Catholic Reporter*, January 21, 2005.

38. Bujo, "Morality for the Problem of AIDS."

39. Downing, "African Perspective on AIDS."

40. Ibid.

VI

THE CHRISTIAN PERSPECTIVE

Debates over HIV/AIDS prevention sometimes devolve into acrimonious disagreement. The emotional sensitivity of the subject indicates that the questions are not solely scientific, but moral, philosophical, and ideological as well.

Competing Visions of the Human Person and Sexuality

Everyone dedicated to the fight against AIDS wants to see fewer people contract the AIDS virus and fewer people suffer its effects. But many are guided by assumptions ingrained within our Western culture that are often not recognized, let alone questioned. Many in modern Western societies find it difficult to grasp the Church's position on sexual morality, especially with respect to contraception, condoms, and HIV. The prohibition of contraception is the "one doctrine the world loves to hate," wrote Mary Eberstadt in her 2008 article "The Vindication of *Humanae vitae*," even though the predictions in the 1968 encyclical about the destructive social consequences of widespread contraception have plainly materialized. For many people even today, the teaching "simply defies understanding"; Eberstadt notes the prevailing mindset: "A ban on condoms when there's a risk of contracting AIDS? Beneath contempt."[1]

The ban is "contemptible," because condom use is mere common sense to those who hold that there are no moral grounds, with the exception of coercion, for limiting sexual activity to marriage. There is broad cultural and legal approval in the modern West for sexual behavior in any context as long as it is consensual. Whether or not sexual activity is situated before, within, or outside of marriage is of no concern to the AIDS Establishment. They may at times counsel against multiple concurrent partnerships because it invites disease, but the objection is a matter of prudence, not moral principle.[2]

In the name of preserving health, the AIDS Establishment emphasizes the pseudo-science of risk reduction. Evidence of its limitations and even its failure erodes this high ground they have claimed for themselves, and thus threatens the underlying sexual liberation project—which is what ultimately propels it. At the end of the day, "Western opinion makers and the media really want the Church to approve of extramarital sex, which is against the religious faith and traditional cultural values shared by millions throughout the world."[3]

This explains why they so desperately want risk reduction strategies to succeed. It also explains why the Church is frequently characterized as being opposed to science and labeled pejoratively as "dogmatic." In this way the Church and its teaching have been dismissed as irrelevant to *real* HIV/AIDS prevention.

This charge does not stand up to scrutiny, but it does call to mind G. K. Chesterton's illuminating observation that "there are only two kinds of people: those who accept dogmas and know it, and those who accept dogmas and don't know it." Each approach to HIV prevention is charged with meaning and expresses an underlying set of values. Any given method "is only proposed by anyone for anyone because there is already an implicit or explicit view of the human person, sexuality, relationships, commitment, self-sacrifice, chastity, and much else besides, at work in the minds of those who develop, those who teach, those who receive, and those who practice the method."[4]

The challenge for Catholics is to articulate the beauty and truth of what the Catholic Church proposes. As Pope John Paul II wrote in *Love and Responsibility*, long before becoming Pope, it is necessary to "validate the 'rules,'" since all human beings, in attempting to integrate sexuality into their personhood, may have "greater difficulties in practice than in theory." The task of the teacher or spiritual director, then, "is not only to command or forbid but to justify, to interpret, to explain."[5] It is necessary to engage the culture, not primarily through technical discourse and debate, but through witnessing to deeper human realities and aspirations. This is no small task, since the Church diverges with the AIDS Establishment not over "science" but over "irreconcilable concepts of the human person and of human sexuality."[6]

The positions of the Church are plainly laid out for all to see. But what exactly is the underlying philosophical foundation of the approaches favored by the AIDS Establishment? The short answer is: a lethal mix of utilitarianism, individualism, and relativism—utilitarianism, in which "no action is ever right or wrong as such," but is only to be evaluated by its consequences;[7] a complementary individualism in which the "right" to unrestrained sexual activity trumps the rights of others, the common good, and the truth; a relativism which subordinates truth to impersonal utilitarian calculations and to the "anything goes" creed of the Western sexual revolution.

Allegiance to these strains of thought, the ultimate rationale for the AIDS Establishment's HIV prevention policy, has made confronting the attitudes and actual behaviors that drive the HIV epidemic almost unthinkable. Yet scrutiny of that mentality and its consequences has been exceedingly rare.

On the other hand, scathing criticism of the Church, on putative "scientific" grounds, has been routine. Some strongly reject the Catholic Church's concept of human sexuality, for example, as if their own views were neutral. Some accused John Paul II of responsibility for AIDS deaths in Africa, because he did not actively promote condoms or change the Church's teachings on sexual morality. In 2005, Nicholas Kristof wrote in the *New*

York Times that "the Vatican's ban on condoms has cost many hundreds of thousands of lives from AIDS," making it one of "its most tragic mistakes in the first two millennia of [the Church's] history."[8] Shortly after the Pontiff's death, a story in the influential English weekly *New Statesman* bluntly stated that "the Pope probably contributed more to the continental spread of the disease than the trucking industry and prostitution combined."[9] Some have suggested that the Vatican could be accused of "crimes against humanity."[10]

The Ideological Assumptions of Global Health Bodies

Where can one go to find an articulation of the ideological assumptions of the AIDS Establishment, including its claim to the truth about humanity—questions which by definition are beyond the reach of science? For the most part, we have to read between the lines. In his remarks for World AIDS Day in 2006, Kofi Annan, secretary-general of the United Nations, vaguely referred to the need to "understand that real manhood means protecting others from risk," meaning that condom use should be synonymous with an enlightened sense of responsible manhood.[11]

Occasionally, however, someone throws cautious ambiguity to the wind and reveals his ideological orientation and agenda more explicitly. In a 2002 speech to the World Bank, Peter Piot, executive director of UNAIDS, claimed that "above all, every community and every country needs to *rewrite the rules* of how it deals with those sensitive issues at the heart of the epidemic—sex, adultery, homosexuality, prostitution, drug use, blood sales, rape, stigma, gender, inequality."[12]

Why do that? Piot cannot say how "the rules" are responsible for HIV transmission, or how doing away with the rules (which are associated with health and well-being) would reduce the epidemic. He cannot say how the rules supposedly make perfect compliance with risk reduction measures impossible—especially if people disregard the rules to begin with. One thing is clear, however: he regards traditional notions of morality as the problem to be overcome. By this twisted but far too common reasoning, if people do not act safely, or if they do but still get AIDS, then traditional morality can always be implicated as the culprit.

Like many in the AIDS Establishment, Piot seeks to jettison traditional morality in its entirety and supplant it with the code of "safety": if you act safely, you act responsibly and do well. There is no place for any other judgments. This ideological pursuit drives Piot, remarkably, to shift responsibility for the disease's transmission from inherently risky behaviors themselves to the "problem" of moral norms. It is a breathtaking display of rhetorical sleight of hand in the finest tradition of the Sophists.

In asserting that we can "rewrite the rules," Piot abandons a notion of truth in favor of the deceptive oppression of relativism, and reduces human freedom to license: personal "freedom" to engage in any sort of behavior. This concept of personal freedom is threatened by any idea of fixed truths and moral norms. It also removes the person from the ties of human relationships. It reflects an impoverished idea of the human person which fails to respect the dignity, aspirations, responsibilities, and ultimate destiny of oneself and others. Sadly, this view informs much HIV prevention policy, with disastrous consequences for the lives of individual human beings.

The breathless appeal to "rewrite the rules" offers an example of what John Paul II described in his 1994 *Letter to Families* as "certain modern cultural agendas" that "'play on man's weaknesses" and lead paradoxically to enslavement rather than liberation.[13] The modern cultural agendas do so by removing the requirements of love from human sexuality, leading to "a man's and a woman's mutual 'use' of each other." This pursuit of the mere satisfaction of sexual appetite "makes persons slaves to their weaknesses."[14] One practical effect of these agendas is seen in the inability of some in the public health community to believe that people can control their sexual behavior, with the result that they emphasize technical solutions, such as the widespread use of condoms (the C strategy), and resist promoting abstinence and fidelity (the A and B strategies), regardless of the evidence.

This is a deeply condescending view, even if it is shrouded in humanitarian rhetoric and rights-based language.

Piot's representative plea to rewrite the rules, fueled by a fierce, modern form of individualism that is prevalent in the West, runs counter to what most people can grasp intuitively and know through reason, and sometimes through painful experience. Self-assertion, in the form of the pursuit of pleasure and power, leads people away from their own fulfillment rather than toward it. George Cardinal Pell of Sydney described this paradox in a 2009 Oxford address: "The possibilities of happiness are greatly restricted by the lovelessness, fear and despair that the assertion of the autonomous self against others usually leaves in its wake."[15] The antidote to self-seeking is proposed by the Church: "Man can fully discover his true self only in a sincere giving of himself."[16]

Despite the fact that values and norms are widely recognized as strong influences on individual behavior, Piot's plea to "rewrite the rules" expresses a desire to do away with them altogether, or at least to fashion them according to a subjective and unbalanced understanding of the human person. In *Veritatis splendor*, John Paul II diagnosed this tendency as "the attempt to adapt the moral norm to one's own capacities and personal interests, and [to reject] the very idea of a norm."[17]

For the AIDS Establishment, norms relating to sexual behavior are to be jettisoned and replaced by rights, which are exalted above all other values. By this stratagem, the actual behaviors fueling the epidemic are ignored and the Church is decried for "driving the epidemic underground" with its moralizing, as if there would be no AIDS or fewer AIDS cases were it not for the Church's outdated injunctions against condom use. This seems contradictory, if not irrational, as it assumes that people knowingly reject the teaching of the Church on the proper place for sexual behavior (within marriage), but rigidly follow its injunctions against contraception.

To judge from his own remarks for World AIDS Day in 2006, Tony Blair, British prime minister, also did not grasp this contradiction: "The danger is [that] if we have a sort of blanket ban from religious hierarchy saying it's wrong to do it, then you discourage people from doing it in circumstances where they need to protect their lives."[18] The Kenyan Catholic bishops described the inconsistency: "Some would have the Church offer such people advice on how to minimize the destructive consequences of their behavior as if, having rejected the central message of life-giving responsibility, they are likely to heed" any particular advice regarding condom use.[19]

Utilitarianism and the Public Health Approach

The discipline of public health, deeply influenced by contemporary culture, relies heavily on particular schools of thought which dictate particular AIDS prevention policies. Chief among them is utilitarianism, an ethical system known for its intent to achieve the "greatest good for the greatest number." This maxim shapes much modern thinking about complex social issues, even if many are unaware of it. It dominates much public health thinking and drives much HIV prevention policy.

Although it has many strands, utilitarianism rests on the assertion that the value or worth of an act is determined solely by its consequences. In this framework, "morality is reduced to doing what one can to minimize pain and suffering and maximize pleasure and enjoyment."[20] As it applies to HIV prevention policy, the objective becomes seeking to maximize the good of sexual pleasure while minimizing the pain of AIDS. Delaying sexual activity or reducing the number of sexual partners would (it is thought) reduce the net amount of sexual pleasure. Yet contracting HIV is an undesirable consequence of seeking maximum sexual pleasure, so all technical remedies short of an actual shift in behavior are enlisted to reduce the risk of infection—even though they cannot eliminate it.

Thus, when Piot proclaims that AIDS obliges every community to "rewrite the rules" related to sexual practices responsible for HIV transmission, he exemplifies the desire to usher in a utilitarian utopia in which the greatest number achieve the greatest sexual pleasure with the fewest negative consequences.

Utilitarianism "displaces traditional morality's focus on intelligible goods—the integrity of the bodily and spiritual person, fidelity, human life, marriage itself—and makes way for a permissive new morality regarding sex, [and] marriage."[21] In eschewing considerations of the moral dimensions of human actions, it replaces them with the individual's own claims and preferences. Having denied and rejected objective moral and philosophical truths, it can advance no internally consistent or coherent rationale for limiting sexual partnerships, and thus tends to yield only *risk reduction* interventions: condoms, treatment for sexually transmitted infections, and voluntary counseling and testing. Inasmuch as these measures are employed to help achieve the greatest good (read: pleasure) for the greatest number, they are quintessentially utilitarian.

Public health officials would not ordinarily be content to downgrade the role of primary behavior change and rely so heavily on mere risk reduction measures. They aggressively promote behavior change for other major health issues such as smoking, obesity, and a sedentary life-style. They recommend quitting smoking, not only recourse to filtered cigarettes; reduction of food intake, and not simply cholesterol-lowering medications; exercise, not merely antihypertensive drugs. In each case they widely advocate the optimal course of action: primary behavior change. The reluctance to do likewise for HIV/AIDS is striking. Furthermore, why are they so principled in aggressively advocating the optimal prevention measures for other infectious diseases, such as SARS, bird flu, polio, and Guinea worm disease, but reluctant to do so for HIV?

Unfortunately, HIV risk reduction measures also serve to facilitate the use and exploitation of one person by another. Utilitarianism, as the name itself implies, allows for just such use of others to serve one's own ends, whether those persons are laborers or lovers.[22] In it, "woman can become an object for man, children a hindrance to parents."[23]

The eminent Canadian philosopher Charles Taylor, in his book *A Secular Age*, described utilitarianism as one of the "theories which deny the human potentiality for moral ascent"; indeed, he referred to it as one of the "crasser variants of Enlightenment secularism."[24] This goes a long way toward explaining the view of the AIDS Establishment that people are not capable of changing their behavior, and the positive depiction of the meretricious in its anti-AIDS campaigns.

It is not only the Church that articulates a vigorous and rational critique of utilitarianism. Influential voices in the contemporary secular world, such as that of sociologist Robert Bellah at the University of California at Berkeley, have likewise lamented "the sombre utilitarianism" in which "the Other becomes an *instrument* to one's self-fulfillment; if they obstruct it or lose attraction or stop fulfilling the needs of the self, they are discarded."[25]

The principal risk reduction approaches to the African AIDS epidemic have failed and in the process have compounded rather than reduced human suffering. Aside from disease, the suffering includes less measurable but no less real emotional anguish. Indeed, people suffer from any number of real but often overlooked consequences of the misuse of sexuality that "are hidden in the hearts of men and women like painful, fresh wounds."[26] These burdensome inner wounds from sexual experiences may afflict a person even in the absence of a sexually transmitted infection, but they are rarely, if ever, factored into public campaigns against AIDS.

These kinds of wounds prompted UCLA psychiatrist Dr. Miriam Grossman to write *Unprotected*, her 2006 book in which she described the emotional and psychological suffering that American students experience as a result of casual sexual encounters. She felt it necessary to publish her book anonymously at first, since she takes aim at the narrow but powerfully entrenched safe-sex approach—the C (risk reduction) strategy—sanctioned by authorities on college campuses. Some college administrators evidently have much in common with the AIDS Establishment, as they both bankroll and emphasize an approach which condones or even glorifies casual encounters while ignoring the havoc that it wreaks on the whole human person.

As we have seen, the risk reduction interventions based on a utilitarian calculus, which have long formed the backbone of HIV prevention policy, have not minimized the damage done by this disease and by other very real, internal wounds, but have resulted instead in a greater prevalence of disease and suffering. The risk reduction approaches represent—and perpetuate—what John Paul II described as "a civilization of 'things' and not of 'persons,' a civilization in which persons are used the same way as things are used."[27] The way to counteract the utilitarian ethic is to foster a profound respect for the dignity of the human person. In a word, its polar opposite is found in love.

Love Counters the Utilitarian Mentality

Despite the fact that the vast majority of global infections occur through heterosexual contact, we hear very little about love—or about the respect for other people as integral human persons, and the responsibility to others, which by definition goes along with love. Such messages from the AIDS Establishment are scarce. The conversation is conducted instead in purely physical and technical terms, reflecting an "utterly materialistic conception of man."[28] Indeed, no public health approach even comes close to what Pope John Paul II suggested should be the main objective of sexual education (of which there is a great need): "to create the conviction that 'the other person is more important than I.'"[29]

In the final analysis, then, the contrasting approaches to HIV prevention differ not on scientific grounds, but because they are informed by competing visions of the human person. This is extremely important today, since the definition of the human person itself is up for grabs; as Cardinal Pell suggests, it ultimately "depends on which understanding of love and sexuality prevails in the culture."[30]

These competing visions lead to diverging convictions over how best to apply science, particularly to an epidemic fueled by human behavior. The AIDS Establishment has limited itself mainly to biomedical approaches to reduce the risk of HIV transmission: promoting condom use, voluntary counseling and testing, and treatment of other sexually transmitted infections but not promoting abstinence and fidelity. Since the risk reduction approach has not produced the intended results—it has not reduced HIV prevalence—we suspect that it maintains its privileged position not because of its efficacy but at least in part because its proponents want to maintain their own vision of the human person, freedom, and sexuality.

The Church, on the other hand, welcomes the developments of science and technology but insists that they be applied toward the authentic service of the human person. The Church has consistently called on the world of science to further its contributions in the fight against AIDS—for instance, in the development of medical treatments. The Church affirms the priority of ethics over technology, however, and proposes that "advances in technology demand a proportional development of morals and ethics," even if, in our present age, the latter development "seems unfortunately to be always left behind."[31] There is no inherent conflict between science and Christianity. When a conflict appears to arise (as when the *Lancet* or *New York Times* editorialized about Pope Benedict's comments on condoms), it is invariably a conflict between a philosophy held by some scientists (and others) and the tenets of Christianity.

The Church rejects certain approaches to HIV prevention, not primarily because of the imperfect nature of the protection they provide, but on legitimate moral grounds—because the Church takes seriously the moral dimensions inherent in human and sexual behavior. As articulated in *Fides et ratio*, the encyclical by John Paul II on the relationship between faith and reason, the Church challenges the premise that "if something is technically possible it is therefore morally admissible."[32] For instance, it is possible to have sexual relations with someone other than one's spouse and, in using a condom on a given single encounter, to reduce the likelihood of contracting HIV. It might likewise be theoretically "safer" to adopt a strategy of engaging in serial monogamy over time as opposed to having multiple concurrent partnerships.

But in either case, Christian communities would not condone the underlying behavior. "Doing something wrong might be safer with a condom, but safety doesn't make the act right. The Church cannot encourage 'safer' without suggesting that it is somehow right."[33] Taking a truly scientific view entails much more than merely applying technology to preventing the spread of a virus which is passed from person to person by specific—and avoidable—human behaviors: it means directing public health strategies and the use of technologies to a higher view of the human person and of human dignity.

Furthermore, love is not unscientific; indeed, it may be considered a higher science. St. Thérèse of Lisieux wrote in her autobiography about her strong desire to live by what she described as the "science of love," which proved to be her distinct vocation.[34] John Paul II would later say that "love therefore is the fundamental and innate vocation of every human being."[35]

In Dostoevksy's *The Brothers Karamazov*, Father Zossima uses the same metaphor when trying to console a "lady of little faith." He first advises her not to be frightened at her own faintheartedness in attaining love, and then gently points out that love in action is harsh compared to love in dreams. "Active love is labor and fortitude, and for some people too, perhaps, a complete science."[36] Dorothy Day, a social justice advocate and the founder of the Catholic Worker Movement, who is commonly associated with "progressive" positions on social issues, was also deeply influenced by the formula of St. Thérèse. Day wrote that "love is a science, a knowledge, and we lack it."[37] How unfortunate and misguided it is to equate science with risk reduction and to miss out on the science of love.

In *Love and Responsibility,* John Paul II wrote that "only love can preclude the use of one person by another."[38] In contrast, the dominant public health approach focuses exclusively on physical factors and rules out the essential consideration of what it means to love others. In this way it advances utilitarian, materialistic, and dualistic notions of the human person and human sexuality. Yet, as so many people throughout the world intuitively grasp, that is "unscientific," reflecting an inadequate understanding of human nature. A human person is "a unity comprised of physical, emotional, intellectual, and spiritual elements."[39]

Pope Benedict's recent encyclical *Deus caritas est* ("God Is Love") counters the materialistic approach to sexuality by reminding us that a human being is "a unified creature composed of body and soul," that love is characterized by "exclusivity," and that love has a quality of permanence over time.[40] The prevailing public health approach admits no limits or boundaries to the expression of sexuality, whereas the Church proposes that it is precisely within the boundaries of marriage that sexuality finds its intended expression. In this way, "love is indeed 'ecstasy,' not in the sense of a moment of intoxication, but rather as a journey, an ongoing exodus out of the closed inward-looking self towards its liberation through self-giving."[41]

Isn't this love the "scientific" discipline that is both most neglected and most relevant to the prevention of a disease whose main source of transmission is by sexual contact, often through multiple partnerships? Couldn't it be more readily explored and proposed by people in all walks of life to counteract the primary source of HIV transmission?

Although Peter Piot's exhortation to "rewrite the rules" for sexual behavior was probably meant to be inspiring, it fails to connect with what is stamped on the human heart, and thus has no real staying power. Decades into the sexual revolution, it is actually a rather dull rallying cry. Its banality comes into full relief when placed next to the truth articulated by Pope John Paul II: "Man cannot live without love. He remains a being that is incomprehensible for himself; his life is senseless if love is not revealed to him, if he does not encounter love, if he does not experience it and make it his own, if he does not participate intimately in it."[42]

This may sound radically idealistic—especially as applied to the AIDS epidemic—but that does not mean that it is not true and even crucial for true human happiness. One colleague, long active in the fight against AIDS in Malawi, described its relevance with the following analogy: "Ideals are like the stars: we may not reach them, but we set our course by them." By its exclusion of love and by its emphasis on risk reduction messages, the dominant approach of the AIDS Establishment sets a philosophical (not scientific) course which is at least partially to blame for our present predicament. So emphasizing love and sound moral approaches to the problems posed by AIDS is of immense, and indeed fundamental, *practical* importance.

The Christian concept of love, entailing as it does an element of sacrifice, is demanding, and it stands diametrically opposed to the many superficial, prevailing notions of love. Challenging as it is, all people—and especially the young—have a yearning and a special capacity to embrace this countercultural "science of love," since it has the intrinsic and eternal appeal of truth.[43]

Truth Liberates the Human Person

The adoption of a utilitarian ethic as the guiding principle for HIV prevention is greatly facilitated by the reigning cultural acceptance of moral relativism. Modern Western cultures have largely replaced confidence in "the enduring absoluteness of any moral value" with the belief that "freedom alone, uprooted from any objectivity, is left to decide by itself what is good and what is evil."[44] In relativistic cultures which contest the truth and refuse to judge between rival conceptions of such basic realities as love, freedom, and the human person, each individual merely evaluates these matters to suit himself. The result is not liberation but rudderless solipsism, a "crisis of truth," as John Paul II described it in *Veritatis splendor,* which ultimately "plung[es] the human person into situations of gradual self-destruction."[45]

Truth is often seen today as cold, rigid, uncaring, and significantly at odds with love, even though, as Pope Benedict explained in his book *Truth and Tolerance,* "truth and Love are identical."[46] But we have a deep-seated, all-too-human tendency to recoil from the truth. Even in pre-Christian times, Plato remarked that men "prefer themselves to the truth."[47]

Why should this be so? Australian Bishop Anthony Fisher, O.P., points out that

> truth often threatens, interrogates, cuts us to the quick: regarding our unjust social structures, institutions, policies; our own long-ingrained and firmly held mis-information, prejudices, ideologies; our own inhumane behaviour, bad ways of relating, self-centredness. Truth tells us that we are very gifted, skilled and often generous people. But it can have harsh things to say about how we use our gifts and privilege, our degrees and qualifications, how carefully confined is our generosity. Truth demands a rethink, an intellectual, moral and personal conversion. It is not just because *veritas* is so hard to capture and communicate, but also because it is so subversive, so seditious, so profoundly disturbing, that we are so often resistant.[48]

Just as a holy person's exemplary life inspires us to be better while serving as an implicit reproach to our moments of mediocrity, speaking about truth, no matter how politely, implies that there *is* a right and a wrong. Since we are all imperfect and fall short of the mark, the mere reminder of objective truth disconcerts everyone from time to time. It cuts us to the quick.

The Church and the AIDS Establishment disagree sharply on what it means to reason in the first place. The Church proposes that there are objective moral and philosophical truths about the human person and human sexuality which require that sexual relationships be reserved for marriage. "Chastity is rooted in the deep respect for the other person, who should never be used as a means merely to satisfy one's sexual desires."[49] And although chastity is related to the human passions, St. Thomas Aquinas described it as keeping conduct under the control of reason.

To acknowledge these truths is not to say that they are always easy to recognize or put perfectly into practice. Living chastely challenges, even as it frees a person from the sometimes capricious impulses of our human appetites by recalling the need to treat oneself and others with respect, and not as mere instruments of sexual satisfaction. Chastity helps a person lead a well-integrated life, and is essential for human fulfillment. Without it, discord and turmoil proliferate.

This view also squares with the teachings of great pre-Christian philosophers such as Plato and Aristotle. In refuting the hedonistic pragmatism proposed by their contemporaries, they, along with many others writers of antiquity and writers in the Jewish tradition, recognized that sexual promiscuity damages the wholeness and well-being of a person.[50] This is important, because the

AIDS Establishment claims that its view of "liberated" human sexuality is based definitively on reason, and consequently that opposing views must simply originate in an unreasoned faith.[51]

Chastity is not an external or arbitrary constraint, but an authentic service of the human person, who is capable of self-control and thus of truly giving his or her entire self in freedom. This liberating moral vision has an internal coherence and consistency that is accessible to reason—for believers and nonbelievers alike.

What the Church proposes as authentic liberation, however, the AIDS Establishment perceives as threat. The Church's insistence that there are healthy limits (for the individual and for the community) to sexual expression directly clashes with the radical individualism at the heart of the sexual revolution, in which the individual's pursuit of sexual pleasure take precedence over the claims of others, the family, and the common good of society.

Christianity sees that human sexuality has transcendental importance for two reasons: not only is it the means for mutual and total giving (gift of body and gift of self) between a man and a woman who love each other, but it can also give rise to the life of a new human being. Men and women, participating freely and generously in the creative work of God, bring forth new human life, created in the image and likeness of God and called to eternal life. These are facets of a good that is so great that the Church zealously safeguards it against anything that could undermine the profound significance of human sexuality. The defense of human life in every possible respect is the fruit of the Christian understanding of human nature and the intrinsic value of each person. The Church cannot renounce her defense of life, or the sanctity of marriage, without undermining herself. These truths must be upheld despite contrary or opposing cultural trends.

A person may adopt any number of technical strategies to reduce the risk of HIV infection, but they do not supplant the inherently moral dimensions of sexual behavior. "The Church does not teach a different sexual morality even when and where AIDS poses no danger."[52] Even if the condom's track record were not so spotty, the central issue in discouraging particular behaviors is not the risk of HIV but the lack of chastity. "But this teaching is not easy for 'the world,' including the media, to understand, much less accept."[53] In bearing witness to this truth, Catholics should not fear hostility or unpopularity, but should avoid "any compromise or ambiguity which might conform [them] to the world's ways of thinking."[54] In fact, they are likely to find many people who, while not belonging to the Catholic fold, nonetheless hold a rational commitment to promoting abstinence and fidelity "unapologetically as a modern and relevant public health message."[55]

Even within the Church, however, some lack confidence in the truth. Some commentators, for instance, set up a false dilemma by pitting notions of compassion or mercy (seen as good) against morality (seen as bad), obscuring the fact that morality is an instrument of authentic liberation because it reflects the truth about the human person. They forget that it is a spiritual work of mercy to point out gently and charitably behaviors that are wrong in hopes of leading a person to health and wholeness.

During a recent visit to an exemplary AIDS program in a Latin American country, we spent some time with highly competent and compassionate religious caregivers. Their witness, dedication, and care for those stricken with AIDS (among others) was truly something to behold and to admire. When the conversation turned from caregiving to prevention, however, they posed a question that highlighted a puzzling conceptual and moral dichotomy: How can the American relief effort (PEPFAR) justify its ABC approach to prevention? Implicit in their question was the unmistakable view that since condoms are capable of reducing the risk of HIV transmission, they must therefore be the first line of defense, making abstinence and fidelity counterproductive distractions.

They regarded the promotion of A and B not as the implementation of Catholic teaching or as a legitimate and plausible approach to the issue, but as "fundamentalism." They quickly added that while the promotion of A and B might be good for the middle class or the well-off, it was just not realistic for the poor. Their view is not easily dismissed, especially since they are dedicated people who minister day in and day out to people living with entirely different physical, psychological, and emotional horizons from ours.

This exchange, and other similar experiences, promoted much reflection, specifically on how such obviously committed people, responding courageously to the Gospel call to care for the sick, could discount other Gospel challenges. Perhaps the best means of explaining this dichotomy can be found in remarks made by Pope Benedict to the Swiss Catholic bishops in 2006.

The Pope suggested that morality in our day is essentially "split in two." Many have a difficult time with the morality that the Church proclaims, but seem to latch onto one dimension, like social justice, as if it were the whole, while leaving out others, like the morality of marriage and family life. The tendency of many to reject ethical considerations with respect to the prevention of HIV, but to embrace ethical directives when the issue is anti-discrimination or access to medications, is entirely emblematic of this "bifurcated" sense of morality. Pope Benedict believes that "we must commit ourselves to reconnecting these two parts of morality and to making it clear that they must be inseparably united."[56]

Thus, part of the challenge of responding to AIDS is presenting both "sides" together with conviction. Doing so would save many from contracting the disease and soothe many who are already afflicted. The Ethiopian Catholic bishops, in their pastoral letter on AIDS, put it in the following terms:

> We sense that the reality of HIV/AIDS presents, in an acute and pressing way, both a great need and an opportunity to articulate the Gospel in its entirety. While fully articulating and fully living out the Gospel is always a challenge, doing so in reference to issues related to HIV/AIDS entails a delicate balance, for in

dealing with the primary cause of HIV transmission, we must deal with issues of morality, respect for self and others, of proper formation of consciences, of just interpersonal relationships, of true love and strengthening family life; in dealing with the effects of HIV and AIDS, we must embrace the need to care for the sick, withhold judgment, provide hope and material support to those in need, promote reconciliation, comfort the bereaved, and care for orphans. We believe that [all] of these responses to HIV/AIDS, rooted in the Gospels, must be wholeheartedly advanced together.[57]

Nonetheless, the impulse to try to minimize harm is real and understandable. Yet it masks a danger that is not readily apparent, though it is worth pausing to consider. Aside from the pragmatic limitations of risk reduction policies in practice, Pope John Paul II suggested that, as a matter of institutionalized policy,

so-called "safe sex," which is touted by the "civilization of technology," is actually, in the view of the overall requirements of the person, radically not safe, indeed it is extremely dangerous. It endangers both the person and the family. And what is this danger? It is the loss of the truth about one's own self and about the family, together with the risk of a loss of freedom and consequently a loss of love itself.[58]

Understanding Risk Reduction and Harm Minimization

While in many cases favoring a risk reduction approach is surely motivated by a genuine sense of compassion, adopting such a course ratifies alluring but flawed assumptions and unintentionally facilitates the very sorts of harmful behavior which then need to be remedied. As the Kenyan Catholic bishops have pointed out, "much as Christians want to reach out tolerantly" to those intent on destructive behavior, "we never want to condone, even mplicitly," behavior that is destructive of oneself and others. It would be "a delusion to imagine that 'compassion' can ever be invoked to tolerate death-dealing actions as being normal or acceptable."[59]

Underlying the risk reduction approach favored by the AIDS Establishment is the assumption that condoms must be relied on as damage control, since sexual promiscuity is a given and people are incapable of being faithful, abstaining from sex, listening to reason, or being influenced positively. Bishop Anthony Fisher, O.P., described as "one of the sharpest minds in English-speaking Catholicism," is an expert in bioethics who commands respect across ideological lines.[60] He points out that "the Church has always opposed such a 'harm minimization philosophy' because beginning with 'if you can't' falsely implies that particular behaviors—sexual promiscuity, underage drinking, prostitution, speeding, drug abuse [and others]—are somehow unavoidable."[61]

To presume that the most we can hope for is "damage control" is to subscribe to an impoverished anthropology. In other words, it is to hold an excessively pessimistic view of the human person—one at odds with the Catholic hope in the potential for human beings, with the help of God's grace, to come to know the truth and to choose the good. Rev. Michael Czerny, S.J., director of the African

Jesuit AIDS Network in Nairobi, explained it this way: "To say, 'Do not commit adultery but, if you do, use a condom' is tantamount to saying: 'The Church has no confidence in you to live the good life.'"[62] He went on to suggest that "as public policy, it is to treat people as rapacious ... incapable of anything beyond immediate self-gratification." When it is "imposed by public and international agencies on Africans, it also represents unconscious but abhorrent racism. This is not a route that the Church can take."

The Church's view that all people have the capacity to change stands in conflict with the AIDS Establishment's view that people are powerless victims of passions and circumstance. The entire harm minimization, or risk reduction, approach, however technically sophisticated or bureaucratically cumbersome it comes to be, ultimately depends on this latter, deeply condescending view of the person.

Thus, resorting to risk reduction, as the AIDS Establishment overwhelmingly does, shortchanges the human person. It confirms low expectations about the possibilities of human behavior and tacitly concedes the inevitability of destructive behaviors. Not to acknowledge the ability of young people and adults to respond to messages about abstinence and fidelity in a context that affirms the precious gift of human sexuality is ultimately a disservice.

Public health professionals and "believers" alike owe more to the people and the communities that they serve. We must place greater trust in the human capacity to respond positively to value-based recommendations, to unselfish ideals, however demanding they may sometimes be. The behavioral expressions of love, in abstinence and faithfulness in mutual monogamy, sometimes require effort, but "such efforts ennoble man and are beneficial to the human community."[63]

Capitulating to harmful behavior in the first place may confirm a sense of despair about prospective relationships. Not daring to counsel against it often says more about ourselves (and our desire to fit in) than it does about those souls who are the object of concern, yet who are themselves moral agents capable of change. Failing to hold out hope and resigning ourselves to "harm minimization" places us in a position of perpetual responsibility for minimizing the physical damage of inadvisable actions. Such an approach is emphatically not liberating in any sense of the word.

In fact, Theodore Dalrymple, a self-described atheist and physician who for decades has tended the poor in the slums of modern England, describes such approaches as inherently "infantilizing."[64] Dalrymple, a prolific writer who is highly praised by other journalists, has spent decades observing and documenting the consequences of the bureaucratically entrenched harm minimization strategies on the lives of those he served in the British underclass. He pierces through the ostensibly benevolent facade of these policies in his 2006 book *Romancing Opiates*, in which he is equally effective in documenting the empirical short-comings of such strategies (notably the failure of efforts to reduce the harmful consequences of drug abuse) as he is in dismantling their philosophical framework.

We must not assume that those involved in prostitution or commercial sex work or those tied into larger sexual networks because of multiple partnerships are irretrievably relegated to a life of risk, degradation, exploitation, despair, and disease. How does this assumption serve the yearning of the heart to be fulfilled and not simply gratified, to live and love fully, and not to be an agent or an object of misuse? For those exasperated by the empty pursuit of fleeting pleasure, those wearied by circumstances of degrading vulnerability, or those anxious about the prospects facing them (including the possibility of contracting AIDS), authentic hope for something better is essential. Without hope for another way of life, and the concrete support of a wider community in helping them realize it, such people are much less likely to succeed in avoiding destructive sexual practices.

HIV prevention, dealing as it does with sexuality, cannot be reduced simply to a physical health issue revolving around the management of risk. By its very nature it raises profound spiritual, theological, and anthropological questions, which are by definition value-laden. These questions cannot be answered by resorting to pure technology or by "providing information," but must be engaged at an altogether different level. In fact, there seems to be widespread agreement, after decades of painful experience, that providing "information" about AIDS has all too often merely served as a gateway to risk reduction strategies and has not proved sufficient to achieve actual changes in behavior.

One example from the West will help to illustrate this. Dr Anthony Fauci, director of the National Institute of Allergy and Infectious Diseases (part of the National Institutes of Health) stated in an April 2009 *Washington Post* article that "the annual number of new HIV infections in the United States—about 56,000—has remained fairly constant for more than a decade. That's right, 56,000 people are infected in this country every year. Clearly, our efforts at HIV prevention have been insufficient. Drastic action and new approaches are urgently needed."[65]

In the United States and other Western countries, almost everyone knows about condoms and about AIDS. In particular, members of high-risk populations (where most domestic transmission occurs) are extremely knowledgeable about condoms and could not be more motivated to use them.

Dr. Fauci's statement about the *steady* rate of infection in the United States is thus a major, albeit implicit, concession that mere "information" and available risk reduction measures have not really worked very well domestically, either. Unfortunately, the policy prescriptions that he offered were not drastically different. He called for more vintage risk reduction measures—recourse to new drug modalities and more voluntary counseling and testing. He made no mention of behavior change.

This, along with the examples described earlier from various countries where successful risk avoidance has occurred, suggests that other things—such as common sense, fear, and a desire to live in harmony with spiritual realities and social boundaries—more profoundly influence human behavior than information and calculation.

Risk reduction approaches invariably pay only lip service to the risk avoidance behaviors that would enable people to avoid contracting AIDS, behaviors which also instill a sense of self-confidence and equip them to forge and maintain healthy and fulfilling relationships. The risk reduction strategies quickly revert to the kinds of "information" dissemination and condom promotion models that have been so ineffectual. This is indicative of a serious flaw in the risk reduction approach: it demotes the basic primary-prevention principle of risk avoidance, which should be the mainstay of sound public health policy.[66]

Although the deficiencies of information-based risk reduction models are increasingly recognized, some attempt to turn the tables and insist that A and B do not work. For example, recent, well-publicized studies analyzing results from abstinence-only and abstinence-centered programs in the United States concluded more or less categorically that "abstinence education is not effective," implying that we should not pursue abstinence education in the future.

The results were based on a meta-analysis of several disparate (heterogeneous) studies in which the number of abstinence education sessions varied greatly, from one to several hundred.[67] One could not expect similar behavioral outcomes from such different educational inputs. Grouping such heterogeneous programs together for evaluation does not yield very meaningful results. Furthermore, those receiving the education were very young, and there were inadequate comparisons to alternative programs. These methodological problems suggest that the conclusions are not reliable enough to be used as the bases for any future policy.

But whether those particular programs worked is not the real issue. The real issue is *how* we can convey the right message—the A-and-B message—not whether we should convey it. If a program aiming to prevent gender violence does not succeed, it would be a terrible mistake to conclude that education against gender violence is not effective and should not be pursued. We would instead have to find a way to help this program to succeed or do it better. The message itself remains valid.

Furthermore, if some increases in risk avoidance behaviors (A and B) in Africa occurred spontaneously—that is, independent of any particular program, as would be expected to be the case—the epidemiological impact remains just as significant. And the A and B messages themselves will always remain good and valid ones to convey.

As we have indicated, HIV prevention by definition deals with value-laden concepts. The whole truth is the best we can give to those in danger of contracting AIDS to help them make better and healthier choices. But we should enable them to make the best choices, and this includes character education. We cannot just give them information and slogans.[68] We have to help them internalize good values and develop the skills and habits that go along with them.

People have an innate yearning to connect; this is good. The question is how best to channel that yearning so that it is life-giving and fulfilling rather than empty and destructive. Therein too lies the challenge, formidable as it is. To view young people and adults as incapable of restraining their sexual desires, as proponents of the risk reduction approach do, only fuels the despair and restlessness that lead to great harm. On the other hand, reminders that no amount of "safe sex" can ever satisfy our deepest desires, that we are made for the kind of "science of love" described earlier, can provide hope and meaning. We are created for more than just the satisfaction of our appetites.

Thus, the Christian message of chastity is one not of repression, but rather of fulfillment and liberation. It is an invitation to experience something greater, something more truly satisfying than mere sexual pleasure. It is a radical yes—an affirmation, and not a senseless collection of prohibitions. It is amazing the challenges to which people are capable of rising, the life-giving choices they can make, even in difficult situations. No matter where people have been, they can still attain freedom and integrity.

Difficult Decisions for Discordant Couples

Although the term "discordant couple" is now in vogue to describe couples in which one partner is infected with HIV and the other is not, it is also vague. It originally referred to married couples but quickly began to refer, in common usage, to any two people of differing HIV status involved in an ongoing sexual relationship. The technical features of risk reduction strategies apply to partners regardless of marital status, but the ambiguity of the term "discordant couple" blurs a central moral distinction.

Another way to think of it is that every time an additional person becomes infected with HIV through sexual contact, the infection is, by definition, a product of a discordant couple relationship—even though, as Sister Alison Munro, O.P., the AIDS coordinator of the Southern African Catholic Bishops Conference, has noted, "many people live in relationships that are far from permanent, very tenuous often in fact."[69] Marriage rates are very low at the epicenter of the epidemic in southern Africa where, as we have described, multiple and concurrent partnerships account for much of the HIV transmission. A very slim percentage of overall HIV transmission is thus attributable to the activity of HIV-discordant married couples.

It would take an entire volume to treat this issue of discordant couples properly and adequately. We do, however, offer a few brief comments, since the issue is often raised as a pretext for dismissing the relevance of abstinence and fidelity, even as a general HIV prevention strategy. After all, what can advocates of A and B, and the opponents of C, say about discordant couples? The issue seems prima facie to demand a technical solution.

The implicit assumption here is that since we are talking about a couple—as opposed to people in any sporadic sexual encounter—it is particularly unreasonable to presume that the persons involved would evaluate their sexual behavior in a new light. As we have shown, abstinence and fidelity are routinely portrayed by the AIDS Establishment as unrealistic and ineffective to begin with. The A option for couples is thus seen as an oxymoron. They are couples, "they are going to do it anyway." And HIV could be transmitted. Seen through this lens—with an established presumption that sexual behavior will persist no matter what—mere moral considerations, such as whether the couple is married or not and whether or not married couples may rightly use condoms, appear to be of remote secondary importance. In fact, these objective moral considerations are sometimes portrayed as inhumane—as an impediment to the ethical imperative to safeguard life.

While this attitude can, of course, parallel the view of the AIDS Establishment that sexual behavior in general cannot or should not change even in the midst of an HIV/AIDS epidemic, in this case it may well also proceed from a positive understanding of the value of human intimacy within marriage.

The fact that a fatal infection can be transmitted to a loved one (and possibly offspring) in a loving and life-giving act accentuates the truly tragic dimensions of HIV/AIDS. A discordant married couple responsibly weighing options together would certainly need all possible support, compassion, and wisdom to face such a delicate and painful situation. Given the good of marital intimacy, many jump to the conclusion that in these circumstances, at least, it is downright foolhardy not to resort immediately to condom promotion.

From a technical perspective, however, it is important to recall that, even if used optimally, a condom does not guarantee that an infection will not be passed to a loved one. It is therefore not accurate to describe condoms categorically as a "life-saving prophylactic," as even some theologians do. Condoms can be. They might be. They might not be.

We must not lose sight of what Father Czerny relates from his own extensive pastoral experience with the African Jesuit AIDS Network: several Africans confided in him that "once they tested positive, they made a firm option for abstinence, rather than risk infecting someone else."[70] This is always a "life-saving" option. They, like other people, need support in living chastely and in demonstrating love, affection, and respect to "the other." Rev. Tadeusz Pacholczyk, a leading American ethicist, has eloquently made this appeal, broaching issues that are rarely mentioned in the public discussion focused on technology:

> A husband who has AIDS would never want to subject the wife he loves to a potentially death-dealing act on his part, which is what sexual intercourse could become for them, even while using a condom (which has a failure rate). Would it be a loving act to subject her to the risk of a possibly fatal encounter, even for something as beautiful as conjugal intimacy in marriage? ... Learning to love each other in different and nongenital ways is, in fact, an integral component of every successful and enduring marriage, and an AIDS infection merely brings greater urgency and immediacy to the task.[71]

Furthermore, as we learned from visiting those with vast experience counseling and accompanying discordant couples in several African countries, some couples who chose the C option nonetheless became infected.

No doubt there are counter-examples. Nevertheless, it is clear that all prevention options (A, B, and C) are not equal, even from a purely medical perspective. The three approaches are likewise unequal from an ethical and moral perspective.

Still, many might simply be inclined to advise the technical fix of condom use, if only to try to "make the best" of a bad situation. This inclination is understandable, not simply because nobody wants to see additional HIV infections, but also because it naturally follows from certain modern ethical presuppositions which dominate the field of bioethics today. In such a difficult case, the temptation is to adopt the ethical posture of consequentialism, or its close cousin, proportionalism.

These pervasive modes of ethical reasoning evaluate the rightness of an act solely on the basis of its foreseeable consequences, or the possible good and bad effects of alternatives, and then determine a course of action according to the overall net benefits. This assessment is "made the exclusive criterion of moral judgment, or the criterion for overriding or qualifying other moral judgments."[72] Under the right circumstances, any act could thus be justified by its good consequences or by the bad consequences it might avert.

Applied to HIV prevention, this means justifying condom use, under the circumstances, in order to make one possible bad consequence of the underlying activity—HIV transmission—less likely. The objective qualities of the behavior itself, which pertain to the marital status of the couple and the integrity of the marital act, are pushed aside, and attention is focused single-mindedly on the attempt to achieve the greatest positive and fewest negative consequences from a course of action that has already been chosen. In this way, the intrinsic moral significance of the underlying act itself is superseded by considerations of how to optimally manage the risk of contracting HIV.

Many Catholic ethicists not inaccurately make a distinction: with regard to unmarried persons in particular, the Church objects to sexual activity in the first place, and therefore the Church cannot issue "rules" for behavior that is already immoral. One can make this distinction while simultaneously holding, as many do, that the promotion of condoms in general is quite harmful anyway, precisely because it suggests approval of extramarital behavior and helps facilitate it.

Taking up the specific issue of condom use within marriage, some argue that it is permissible to use condoms to gain the greater good of blocking HIV transmission. Usually they bolster this claim by arguing that the intent in this case is not contraceptive but prophylactic.

One immediate problem, however, is that the "greater good" in this case is to be extracted from an act that is already wrong to begin with. That would invalidate the common attempt to classify it as the "'lesser evil," since it does not meet the traditionally accepted requirements for applying the principle. It may be permissible, provided certain conditions are met, to do a good action even if that action entails a foreseen though unintended bad consequence. But *Veritatis splendor* clarifies that "it is never lawful, even for the gravest reasons, to do evil that good may come of it ... even though the intention is to protect or promote the welfare of an individual, of a family or of society in general."[73]

One of the reasons most often voiced by some theologians for justifying condom use by discordant couples is that HIV/AIDS is *fatal*. They portray condoms as *the* life-saving alternative; if a person takes care to maximize the likelihood of preserving life, then the action may be justified.

Although life-prolonging medical treatments for HIV/AIDS have improved tremendously over the past decade, a cure or a vaccine is not imminent. If or when one becomes widely available, however, would these same theologians then conclude that condom use is no longer justifiable for HIV discordant couples? On the whole, one suspects not. Even if it were no longer fatal in all cases, HIV/AIDS could still well be a source of considerable morbidity and inconvenience—an undesirable consequence, just like any other sexually transmitted infection or even pregnancy.

Indeed, many commentators of the proportionalist and consequentialist persuasion have said as much. They go much further by stressing that the good and proper thing to do (in general and beyond marriage) is to "act responsibly" by seeking to minimize threats to life and health and the possibility of other unwanted outcomes such as pregnancy. After all, since condoms are capable of bestowing on anyone the benefit of reduced risk of transmitting or acquiring a harmful virus—whether the exposure comes through prostitution, casual sex, a stable relationship, or marriage—many adherents of this line of reasoning are hard pressed to articulate why encouraging condom use should be limited to married couples. Or limited to just HIV.[74]

These ethical theories dispense with objective criteria for evaluating actions and leave dizzying difficulties in their place. For starters, would the decision to use condoms in marriage still be right in the event that the hoped-for consequence of averting HIV infection is not achieved? If so, the actual consequence *per se* would not make the action right but rather the calculated intent. Is it then merely the intention to avert disease that constitutes an unassailable ethical position? A person's intent in using condoms could very well be to perpetuate the self-seeking pursuit of sexual pleasure by diminishing the prospects of disease or pregnancy. Alternatively, a person's intent to use condoms might not be to inhibit procreation at all, but rather to prevent disease. This is a more common argument, and it could very well be the case that a person would have this genuine intent. But if the ethical value of an action can be determined solely on the basis of intent, we would be unable to evaluate the ethical quality of condom use (or indeed of *any* other act) unless we knew the intent of each person who uses a condom.[75] What if the intents of the couple are mixed?

The challenging reality is that, any way you slice it, significant ethical problems with these theories remain. Weighing the possible consequences of an act and evaluating the subjective intentions of individuals involved are both *essential* components of responsible ethical deliberation. However, the Church teaches (as most recently articulated in *Veritatis splendor*) that these considerations are "not sufficient for judging the moral quality of a concrete choice." Alone, they are simply "not an adequate method for determining whether the choice of that concrete kind of behavior is ... 'in itself,' morally good or bad, licit or illicit."[76]

For these reasons, the Church emphatically rejects these prevailing theories—consequentialism and proportionalism—which are not grounded in the Catholic moral tradition.[77] Nonetheless, as *Veritatis splendor* goes on to say, these theories have "a certain persuasive force" today.[78] Their influence is nearly universal in secular culture, but they have also made great inroads into the intellectual life of the Church. Proportionalist reasoning on this specific topic of HIV prevention has surfaced in some of the statements of local Church bodies (such as *AIDS: Society in Question* in France and *The Many Faces of AIDS* in the United States), even though Church teaching explicitly rejects it.[79]

These ethical views can sound reasonable at first because they propose what seem to be self-evident solutions. Yet the highly esteemed twentieth-century philosopher Elizabeth Anscombe, who gave consequentialism its name, felt that that theory has "proven to be a profoundly destructive force, not only in ethics considered as a field of academic philosophy, but in the ethical lives of individuals and cultures. The conviction that a little evil may rightly be done for the sake of a greater good, or for the sake of preventing a greater evil, puts human beings on the path to losing their grip on good and evil altogether."[80]

Something other than circumstances, intentions, and consequences is needed to establish the goodness of an act in itself, since they "can never transform an act intrinsically evil by virtue of its object into an act 'subjectively' good or defensible as a choice."[81] The Church thus views the matter from an altogether different vantage point, and insists that the "morality of the human act depends primarily and fundamentally on the 'object'" (the act) itself.[82] Condom use is not countenanced because, considered objectively, it obstructs the procreative dimension of the marital act *and* because it interferes with the unitive dimension. The Church further maintains that there are valid alternatives to the use of condoms.

If health professionals wish to adhere to Catholic teaching, what do they need to consider with regard to condom use by discordant couples?

The overarching consideration which applies to all possible circumstances of any particular couple is that "it is never the role of the Church, or its agencies, pastors or members, to help people do the wrong things more efficiently or safely."[83]

The question then becomes, what are the wrong things? To put it briefly, the wrong things here are sexual activity outside of marriage and condom use (whether strictly contraceptive or not) within marriage. Some, including Bishop Anthony Fisher, have treated the finer points of these moral and philosophical matters in great detail, and with great rigor and pastoral sensitivity.[84]

A Catholic health professional in regular contact with unmarried discordant couples should take the same approach as with other people (even those in high-risk groups), by recommending the optimal course of action—in other words, risk avoidance. That is always an option. This alternative to the present behavioral pattern must always be proposed in every professional encounter with a particular patient, for reasons of health, morality and well-being.

A married discordant couple might, in certain circumstances, wish to consummate their marriage and to conceive a child. The likelihood of passing on the virus in a single act of intercourse is variable, depending on viral load and stage of infection, among other things. In a best-case scenario, when the infected person is fully compliant with antiretroviral medications and other variables line up favorably, the likelihood of HIV transmission during a single act is quite small. Still, this ideal scenario represents the distinct minority of cases in Africa. Nonetheless, some couples may, after careful consideration, and fully aware of the risks, choose to have marital relations.

This is not to suggest that the condom issue needs be ignored or avoided entirely. It would be naive to think that the client would not know about condoms, or that condoms would not surface as a topic of conversation between the patient or client and the health professional. On the contrary, having time to discuss the issue in detail would present an opportunity for the professional to engage the patient in a deeper, more personalized manner.

Here it is important to keep in mind that information about condoms is difficult to convey without sending other signals. Knowledge itself is of course a good, and ignorance a vice. But the line between providing information about a course of action—particularly about its benefits—and tacitly approving it or cooperating with it, quickly becomes blurred. Neutrality—merely being a conduit of information—is an illusion.

This makes resorting to disinterested "information" about condoms morally problematic. However, information about condoms could be presented accurately by the health professional in the context of attempting to dissuade persons from the underlying behavior, "by educating them about the moral and physical dangers of such a course and proposing to them morally and medically preferable options."[85]

The Catholic health professional is essentially responsible for the guidance that he or she gives—for how he or she presents information and alternatives. He or she cannot be held responsible for whatever particular action a client ultimately chooses to take.

Counseling people in such circumstances is certainly a challenge. Some concepts may be difficult to convey and assimilate. Some clients may not be well equipped or well disposed to make adjustments. We recognize that there are many heartbreaking situations with no easy answers. Yet what the Church teaches does not contradict sound health care principles.

Traditional African Values and Culture

We have described how risk reduction strategies have failed to halt the AIDS epidemic. Appeals to the heart, to deeper human aspiration about the meaning of life and human sexuality, have a universal attractiveness: "Although cultural conditions affect men and women of different times and places, the condition of man's heart ... remains the same in every time and place."[86] Furthermore, most traditional cultures (and not only those in the Christian tradition) hold marriage, family life, abstinence, and fidelity as norms that are both possible and desirable. "In traditional societies, various practices helped promote good behavior, and to maintain faithfulness and integrity in marriage: girls and young women protect their virginity; young men control their sexual desires."[87] In Kenya, as the Kenyan bishops have pointed out, a "virgin bride was much esteemed in almost all African cultures, and her family loaded with gifts ... so when the Church condemns premarital and extramarital sex, it is neither asking for the impossible nor proposing something altogether contrary to our traditions."[88]

In the Mpumalanga province of South Africa, not far from the Swaziland border, we listened to an elderly Zulu woman, active as a nurse among people with AIDS, who spoke eloquently of her own experience of those cultural practices designed to protect young women. She told us how, when she was an adolescent, older female relatives took her aside to describe changes that would come with her maturation into womanhood, and how she could find support from others in protecting herself from unwanted advances and premature relationships. She lamented that these customs and practices had largely vanished as a result of rapid modernization and urbanization, but her witness is evidence that they are not beyond the people's consciousness. In fact, Africans themselves have reasonably suggested that "instead of considering these behaviors as old-fashioned, as understood in the West, one should buckle down and study the way of encouraging these practices by giving value to the positive elements of the African culture."[89]

This would seem to form a solid basis for hope. As Pope John Paul II pointed out, "Africa constitutes a real treasure-house of so many authentic human values."[90]

Instead of persisting in imposing an ideological vision that contradicts many of these human values and has proved ineffective anyway, we might again consider the alternatives: "The world must learn to receive from the people of Africa. It is not just material and technical aid that the latter need. They need also to give: their heart, their wisdom, their culture, their sense of man, their sense of God, which are keener than in many others."[91]

The West also desperately needs to retrieve these human values. They were once more routinely instilled, but they have been massively eroded, particularly in recent decades. Many in the modern West, of course, still embrace these values and find in them a source of fulfillment and hope for the future. This would suggest that there is a reservoir of these values within individuals and families, and perhaps even buried in the deep recesses of the collective psyche. But by and large, many modern Westerners are unequipped to mine this rich ore, and they often end up ridiculing it.

Comparisons to other historical eras can sometimes be difficult to make; chastity perhaps has never been "popular" or easy, to be sure. Yet there is something radically askew in modern Western cultures. Elizabeth Anscombe perceived that Western Catholics, in the present day and age, encounter a cultural environment that is even more hostile to chastity than was the "pagan" environment which the first Christians encountered. She put the differences in the following terms: "Christianity taught that 'men ought to be as chaste as pagans thought honest women ought to be'; modernity teaches that 'women need to be as little chaste as pagans thought men need to be.'"[92]

Notes

1. Mary Eberstadt, "The Vindication of *Humanae vitae*," *First Things* 185 (August–September 2008): 35.

2. See Robert George, "A Clash of Orthodoxies," *First Things* 95 (August–September 1999): 33–40; and Michael Czerny, "The Pope and AIDS in Africa: A Human and Spiritual Wake Up Call," *Thinking Faith* (March 25, 2009), http://www.thinkingfaith.org/articles/20090325_1.htm.

3. Czerny, "The Pope and AIDS in Africa."

4. Anthony Fisher, "The Pastoral Application on the Theology of the Body" Centrecare Natural Family Planning Conference, Randwick, Australia, October 23, 2004, http://www.sydney.catholic.org.au/people/bishop_anthony_fisher/addresses/2004/20041023_819.shtml.

5. Karol Wojtyla, *Love and Responsibility* (San Francisco: Ignatius, 1993), 16.

6. John Paul II, *Familiaris consortio* (November 22, 1981), n. 32.

7. Alasdair MacIntyre, *After Virtue: A Study in Moral Theory* (Notre Dame, IN: University of Notre Dame Press, 1981), 15.

8. Nicholas D. Kristof, "The Pope and AIDS," *New York Times*, May 8, 2005.

9. Michela Wrong, "Blood of Innocents on His Hands," *New Statesman*, April 11, 2005.

10. Rosemary Neill, "A Catholic Culture of Death," *Australian*, May 7, 2005.

11. Kofi A. Annan, message on the occasion of World AIDS Day, December 1, 2006, http://data.unaids.org/pub/PressStatement/2006/SG-worldaidsday2006.rev.pdf.

12. Peter Piot, "AIDS: The Need for an Exceptional Response to an Unprecedented Crisis," a Presidential Fellows lecture, November 20, 2003, emphasis added, http://data.unaids.org/Media/Speeches02/Piot_WorldBank_20Nov03_en.pdf.

13. John Paul II, *Letter to Families* (February 2, 1994), n. 13.

14. Ibid., n. 13.

15. George Cardinal Pell, "Varieties of Intolerance: Religious and Secular," Inaugural Hilary Term Lecture, Oxford University Newman Society, March 6, 2009, http://users.ox.ac.uk/~newman/varietiesofintolerance.pdf.

16. Vatican Council II, *Gaudium et spes* (December 7, 1965), n. 24.

17. John Paul II, *Veritatis splendor* (August 6, 1993), n. 105.

18. Ben Russell, "It's Time You Faced Up to AIDS, Tony Blair Tells Church Leaders," *Irish Independent*, December 2, 2006, http://www.independent.ie/national-news/its-time-you-faced-up-to-aids-tony-blair-tells-church-leaders-62659.html.

19. Kenya Catholic Church HIV and AIDS Taskforce, *This We Teach and Do* (Nairobi: Kenya Episcopal Conference—Catholic Secretariat, 2006).

20. Germain Grisez, *The Way of the Lord Jesus*, vol. 3, *Difficult Moral Questions* (Quincy, IL: Franciscan Press, 1997), 80.

21. Ibid.

22. George Weigel, *Witness to Hope: The Biography of Pope John Paul II* (New York: Harper Collins, 1999).

23. John Paul II, *Letter to Families*, n. 13.

24. Charles Taylor, *A Secular Age* (Cambridge, MA: Belknap/Harvard, 2007), 372, 385.

25. Cited in Anthony Fisher, "Moral Theology from Vatican II to John Paul II," lecture to Australian Confraternity of Catholic Clergy National Conference, Galong, New South Wales, Australia, July 14, 1998, 6, original emphasis.

26. John Paul II, *Letter to Families*, n. 14.

27. Ibid., n. 13.

28. Paul VI, *Humanae vitae* (July 25, 1968), n. 23.

29. Wojtyla, *Love and Responsibility*, 274.

30. Pell, "Varieties of Intolerance."

31. John Paul II, *Redemptor Hominis* (March 4, 1979), n. 15.

32. John Paul II, *Fides et ratio* (September 14, 1998), n. 88.

33. Czerny, "The Pope and AIDS in Africa."

34. St. Thérèse of Lisieux, *Story of a Soul*, trans. John Clark (Washington, D.C.: Institute of Carmelite Studies, 2005), 294.

35. John Paul II, *Familiaris consortio*, n. 11.

36. Fyodor Dostoyevsky, *The Brothers Karamazov*, trans. Constance Garnett (New York: Signet Classic, 1999), 66.

37. Robert Ellsberg, ed., *By Little and By Little: The Selected Writings of Dorothy Day* (New York: Knopf, 1983), 189.

38. Wojtyla, *Love and Responsibility*, 30.

39. Anthony Fisher, "Theology of the Body: Love, Life, Sex—The Good News about Sexuality," presented at a seminar of the Australian Council of Natural Family Planning, Sydney, October 10, 2003.

40. Benedict XVI, *Deus caritas est* (December 25, 2006), nn. 5 and 6.

41. Ibid., n. 6.

42. John Paul II, *Redemptor Hominis*, n. 10.

43. Ethiopian Catholic Bishops, "Love As Our Main Tool of Overcoming HIV/AIDS," pastoral letter, Addis Ababa, February 25, 2007.

44. John Paul II, *Veritatis splendor*, n. 84.

45. Ibid., nn. 32 and 84.

46. Benedict XVI, *Truth and Tolerance: Christian Belief and World Religions* (San Francisco: Ignatius, 2004), 231, cited in Basil Meeking, "Proclaim the Truth through Love: A Comment on *Deus caritas est*," *Logos* 10.3 (Summer 2007): 91.

47. Cited in Alice Von Hildebrand, "Why Truth and Charity Are Inseparable," *AD2000* 20.6 (July 2007).

48. Anthony Fisher, speech at the Graduation Mass, University of Notre Dame, Fremantle, Australia, July 16, 2006.

49. Janet Smith, "Chastity," in *Our Sunday Visitor's Encyclopedia of Catholic Doctrine*, ed. Russell Shaw (Huntington, IN: OSV, 1997), 92.

50. See Avery Cardinal Dulles, "Can Philosophy Be Christian?" *First Things* 102 (April 2000): 24–29.

51. See George, "Clash of Orthodoxies."

52. Kenya Catholic Church HIV and AIDS Taskforce, *This We Teach and Do*.

53. Ibid.

54. John Paul II, *Evangelium vitae* (March 25, 1995), n. 82.

55. Leclerc-Madlala, "Behaviours That Drive Our HIV/AIDS Crisis."

56. Benedict XVI, Conclusion of the meeting with the Bishops of Switzerland (November 9, 2006).

57. Ethiopian Catholic Bishops, "Love as Our Main Tool," 33.

58. John Paul II, *Letter to Families*, n. 13.

59. Kenya Catholic Church HIV and AIDS Taskforce, *This We Teach and Do*.

60. See John L. Allen, "The World from Rome," *National Catholic Reporter*, October 31, 2003, http://www.nationalcatholic reporter.org/word/word103103.htm.

61. Anthony Fisher, "The Catholic Church and the Drug Crisis," talk given to the Endeavour Forum at St. Joseph's Hall, Malvern, Australia, February 10, 2000.

62. Czerny, "The Pope and AIDS in Africa."

63. Paul VI, *Humanae vitae*, trans. NC News Service (Boston: Pauline Books and Media, 1968), n. 20.

64. Theodore Dalrymple, *Romancing Opiates* (New York: Encounter Books, 2006), 41.

65. Anthony S. Fauci, "A Policy Cocktail for Fighting HIV," *Washington Post*, April 16, 2009, http://www.washingtonpost. com/wp-dyn/content/article/2009/04/15/AR2009041503040 .html.

66. J. N. Santamaria, "Drug Abuse: The Battle over Harm Minimisation," H. R. Francis Memorial Lecture, May 2003, rev. November 26, 2004, Drug Advisory Council of Australia, http://www.daca.org.au/rehab/BA_santamaria.htm.

67. Jokin de Irala, "Sexual Abstinence Education: What Is the Evidence We Need?" *British Medical Journal*, August 20, 2007, http://www.bmj.com/cgi/eletters/335/7613/248 (2007).

68. Kelly Ladin L'Engle, Jane D. Brown, and Kristin Kenneavy, "The Mass Media Are an Important Context for Adolescents' Sexual Behavior," *Journal of Adolescent Health* 38.3 (2006):186–192.

69. Alison Munro, "Responsibility: The Prevention of HIV/ AIDS," in *Responsibility in a Time of AIDS: A Pastoral Response by Catholic Theologians and AIDS Activists in Southern Africa*, ed. Stuart C. Bate (Pietermaritzburg, South Africa: Cluster Publications, 2003), 32.

70. Czerny, "The Pope and AIDS in Africa."

71. Tadeusz Pacholczyk, "Conundrum with Condoms," *Making Sense Out of Bioethics* column, June 2006, National Catholic Bioethics Center, http://64.105.206.27/NetCommunity/Page .aspx?pid=284.

72. John Finnis, *Fundamentals of Ethics* (Oxford: Clarendon Press, 1984), 86.

73. John Paul II, *Veritatis splendor*, n. 80, citing Paul VI, *Humanae vitae*, n. 14.

74. For a representative example, see Michael Kelly, "The Church as Servant, Teacher and Prophet in Today's HIV/AIDS Crisis," *Jesuit Centre for Theological Reflection* 44 (Second Quarter 2000), http://www.jesuitaids.net/go.aspx?B1=htm/ Church%20as%20Leader.htm&RZ=1&TL=1.

75. David Crawford, "Conjugal Love, Condoms, and HIV/AIDS," *Communio* 33.3 (Fall 2006): 505–512.

76. John Paul II, *Veritatis splendor*, n. 77.

77. Ibid., n. 76.

78. Ibid.

79. Agnė Širinskienė, "Manifestation of Different Ethical Theories in the Content of HIV Prevention" [in Polish], *SOTER: Religijos mokslo žurnalas* 21.49 (2007): 153–162. See also the letter of Josef Cardinal Ratzinger to Archbishop Pio Laghi, Apostolic Pronuncio in the United States, May 29, 1988.

80. Cited in Robert George, "Sweet Reason," review of *Human Life, Action, and Ethics: Essays by G.E.M. Anscombe, First Things* 159 (January 2006): 56–59.

81. John Paul II, *Veritatis splendor*, n. 81.

82. Ibid., n. 78.

83. Anthony Fisher, "Cooperation, Condoms and HIV," Henkels Lecture at the Institute of Bioethics, Franciscan University of Steubenville, Ohio, October 9, 2008, http://www.sydney .catholic.org.au/people/bishop_anthony_fisher/addresses/ 2008/2008109_954.shtml.

84. Ibid.

85. Ibid., n. 6.

86. Christopher West, *Theology of the Body Explained* (Boston: Pauline Books and Media, 2003), 167.

87. Michael Czerny, "AIDS: Africa's Greatest Threat since the Slave Trade," *La Civiltà Cattolica* 3741 (May 6, 2006), http://www .jesuitaids.net/pdf/2006_Czerny_AIDS_Civilta_ENG.pdf.

88. Kenya Catholic Church HIV and AIDS Taskforce, *This We Teach and Do*.

89. Czerny, "AIDS: Africa's Greatest Threat."

90. John Paul II, Address to the diplomatic community in Nairobi (May 7, 1980), n.11.

91. Therese Wilson Favors, "Three Popes Who Came from Africa," *Catholic Review*, April 28, 2005, 30.

92. Cited in Fisher, "Cooperation, Condoms and HIV."

VII

THE PATH TO PROGRESS

Hearing so much about the magnitude of the problem of HIV/AIDS, we could be led to believe that AIDS affects millions of anonymous, faceless people in distant countries. It would be easy to lose sight of the fact that in each case an individual person is confronted with the pain of illness, with emotional anguish, heartache, and alienation, and with the likelihood of an early death. AIDS is affecting beautiful people who are full of life and dreams and plans, who love and are loved by those around them—unique people who are grandmothers, grandfathers, mothers, fathers, daughters, sons, relatives, and friends.

The vast suffering and destruction caused by AIDS and the continuing threat it poses are major human dramas. Consistent with its call to be a Good Samaritan, the Church cares for approximately 27 percent of the people living with HIV/AIDS worldwide, regardless of race, religion, or personal convictions.[1]

Indeed, the Church has a long tradition of caring for the sick and the outcast. The words of St. John of God, who lived in the sixteenth century and is revered as the patron saint of the sick, capture the ethos behind caring for those with distressing diseases like AIDS, especially the poor and rejected among them: "Since our house is open to all, it receives the sick of every kind and condition; the crippled, the disabled, the lepers, mutes, the insane, paralytics, those suffering from scurvy, and those bearing the infirmities of old age, many children, and countless pilgrims and travelers whom we give fire, water, salt and cooking utensils. We ask no payment from anyone, and yet Christ provides for all."[2]

Many with HIV/AIDS also suffer emotionally; indeed, such anguish is often as acute as their physical suffering. For this reason, many very active religious have told us that their work responding to AIDS in Africa has been as much pastoral as it has been clinical. In this sense, AIDS differs from many other diseases. The Church thus strives to accompany those coping with HIV/AIDS to "face the challenge not only of the sickness but also the mistrust of a fearful society that instinctively turns away from them."[3]

Many individuals with HIV/AIDS thirst not only for medicines but for words of encouragement and consolation. Aware of this acute need, the Ethiopian Catholic bishops proclaimed their closeness to people suffering from AIDS in a nationally distributed pastoral letter: "Considering too that our Savior was 'spurned and avoided by men' (Isaiah 53:3), we further recall the promise of the Lord: 'Can a mother forget her infant, be without tenderness for the child of her womb? Even should she forget, I will never forget you' (Isaiah 49:15)."[4]

In each personal circumstance, a compassionate human presence simply cannot be replaced. One American woman we met at a dilapidated Baltimore nursing home had been blinded and crippled by the effects of HIV/AIDS. She struggled with the impersonal and sometimes frightening environment to which her physical immobility confined her. She revealed to us how, particularly while lying awake at night, pangs of regret would settle over her as she recalled the prior turmoil in her life. She did not know where to begin to find relief for that. But she was immensely consoled by Jean Pierre de Caussade's counsel: "To escape the distress caused by regret for the past or fear about the future, this is the rule to follow: leave the past to the infinite mercy of God, the future to His good providence, give the present wholly to His love by being faithful to His grace."[5] This gave her a great sense of hope and soothed her.

The same fidelity to the Gospel which compels the Church to care for the sick also compels it to proclaim the value, importance, and possibility of chastity. The common thread uniting care and prevention is profound respect for the dignity and value of the human person. Christian agencies, and especially Catholic agencies, are joyfully bound to be a witness to the truth about man and to the dignity of every human being as a free and responsible agent, and to the precious gift of sexuality.

Seen in this way, upholding these values is a declaration, particularly to the young, that their lives matter, that their choices matter. It amounts to issuing a hope-filled wake-up call, "telling people that they are all walking around shining like the sun."[6] The Ethiopian Catholic bishops put it like this:

> Your life has meaning and tremendous value! ... The Lord has said, "Before I formed you in the womb, I knew you and consecrated you" (Jeremiah 1:5). We wish to support you in the adventure of learning the meaning of true love and valuing the gift of human sexuality within marriage, to support you in your pursuit of chastity. We urge you to "not let yourself be led astray by those who would ridicule your chastity or your power to control yourselves. The strength of your future married love depends on the strength of your present effort to learn about true love."[7]

The world is in great need of this message, which stands in competition with very powerful if less respectful cultural messages about the human person and sexuality. Culture itself, as a determinant of thoughts, attitudes, and actions, is one but by no means the only factor which influences HIV transmission. Protecting what is good within a culture, modifying what is harmful, and infusing the culture with a sense of authentic human values is thus an important means of protecting people from HIV transmission. The Church would further propose that "the first and fundamental step towards this cultural transformation consists in *forming consciences* with regard to the incomparable and inviolable worth of every human life."[8]

In an August 2006 interview, Pope Benedict XVI indicated that this formation was the key to the entire response to AIDS. A reliance on technical measures without the "formation of the heart" proves fruitless: "If we only teach how to build and to use machines and how to use contraceptives, then we should not be surprised when we find ourselves facing wars and AIDS epidemics."[9]

He also had the opportunity directly to respond to the common misconception that the Church is somehow preoccupied with preserving arcane "rules" over human lives, essentially letting the answer to the question he posed speak for itself:

> So that's the problem: do we really pay so much attention to moral issues? I think—I am more and more convinced after my conversations with the African bishops—that the basic question, if we want to move ahead in this field, is about education, formation. Progress becomes true progress only if it serves the human person and if the human person grows: not only in terms of his or her technical power, but also in his or her moral awareness. I believe that the real problem of our historical moment lies in the imbalance between the incredibly fast growth of our technical power and that of our moral capacity, which has not grown in proportion.

Considering all the evidence, we would hope that all relevant actors would adopt a more sensible approach to HIV prevention that articulates the advantages of avoiding the risk of infection and offers concrete support in doing so. International agencies, Western donors, and medical journals should more willingly welcome the promotion of the A and B strategies as scientifically legitimate. As members and leaders of the scientific community, they have an opportunity to distinguish themselves once again by adherence to objectively sound and medically valid principles of health and well-being. In so doing, they would distinguish themselves from the *zeitgeist* to which they have too often conformed.

Many organizations outside the Catholic Church also favor the A and B messages. The fact that these priorities can be derived from and supplemented by messages of faith, hope, and love fosters a sense of purpose and direction in life. All people of good will can rally around these things (and around respect for self and others), since these principles are supported by science and common sense as well as by faith. It seems reasonable that the work of organizations promoting risk avoidance strategies should be prioritized, whether or not they are rooted in Christian faith.

We would submit that it is here, in the affirmation of well-integrated sexuality, marriage, and family life, the formation of the heart, and the evangelization of culture, that the worlds of Africa and the West may each gain the most in confronting their different but not unrelated physical, cultural, and spiritual pathologies. For every individual person, and for the societies at large, the Church proposes the Gospel, the "good news," with a new urgency, because "the 'new evangelization' is a matter of life and death for the Church and the world."[10]

Pope Benedict has said that the great themes of service animating the Church's response to AIDS—the themes of evangelization and social work—cannot be separated from each other:

> Every now and then … [an] African Bishop will say to me, "If I come to Germany and present social projects, suddenly every door opens. But if I come with a plan for evangelization, I meet with reservations." Clearly some people have the idea that social projects should be urgently undertaken, while anything dealing with God or even the Catholic faith is of limited and lesser urgency. Yet the experience of those Bishops is that evangelisation itself should be foremost, that the God of Jesus Christ must be known, believed in and loved, and that hearts must be converted if progress is to be made on social issues and reconciliation is to begin, and if—for example—AIDS is to be combated by realistically facing its deeper causes and the sick are to be given the loving care they need. Social issues and the Gospel are inseparable. When we bring people only knowledge, ability, technical competence, and tools, we bring them too little.[11]

No doubt the humanitarian application of knowledge and technical know-how has led to tremendous progress in providing treatment to thousands upon thousands of people in Africa. But technical know-how has not managed to curtail the accumulation of new HIV cases. As we have shown, reductions in HIV rates in a handful of African countries are most attributable to changes in behavior, and not to various risk reduction measures. Yet the AIDS Establishment seems intent on redoubling its commitment to the failed philosophy of risk reduction, and to package it as a commitment to science over ideology.

We have shown that risk reduction is a philosophy that places no premium on hope and no confidence in the human capacity to change. And hope for the future is what is needed most—hope to be healed of past traumas, hope to live free of disease, discord, and inner turmoil.[12]

Risk reduction is a natural extension of dominant strains of thought in modern Western cultures—cultures that have over time experienced not only a loss of faith, but also "*a decline or obscuring of the moral sense*," as Pope John Paul II has put it.[13] Approaches that offer much more than risk reduction, ones that hold out a challenging standard to which all may aspire, remind us of that moral sense, which may be why they are often viewed with distrust by the AIDS Establishment.

The philosophy of risk reduction deserves much greater critical scrutiny. We rightly and regularly scrutinize epidemiological evidence in appropriately empirical terms. Evaluating risk reduction as a *philosophy* needs to be approached differently. Since this philosophy, more than anything else, shapes our poorly performing AIDS prevention policies, such scrutiny is long overdue.

Individualism, utilitarianism, and relativism are the tenants which occupy many minds in the West today. As long as public health authorities, which includes the AIDS Establishment, remain wholly committed to these prevailing ideas when addressing lifestyle diseases, fresh approaches will be resisted. Yet there is no good reason why public health leaders or anyone else should remain captive to these elements of Western culture or downplay evidence that questions their wisdom. By virtue of their responsibility and authority, public health authorities should be expected to challenge counterproductive ideas and to more strenuously promote those that truly foster human well-being.

We should, in other words, expect our public health authorities to be not merely another uncritical conduit of the prevailing culture but a firewall against it. Refuge from the emptiness of radical individualism, the impersonal coldness of utilitarianism, and the despair of relativism is simply essential for integral human development today. Although these "isms" are routinely portrayed as innocuous, pragmatic, inclusive, and enlightened, they are in fact deeply hostile to human flourishing.

We need to keep striving to provide ethical means of technical know-how—including the best treatments as well as generous and effective care for those afflicted with HIV and AIDS. But all of us, particularly those threatened by the prospect of HIV transmission, need the protection of better ideas, ideas that reinforce love, hope, and confidence in the inestimable worth of every human being.

The peoples of Africa and the West stand together in their need for just such a firewall. The odds of displacing the prevailing paradigm certainly appear long. But with Africa's willingness to lead, to insist on a hopeful and successful alternative, perhaps we can build it together.

Notes

1. Javier Lozano-Barragán, statement to the Twenty-sixth Special Session of the General Assembly on HIV/AIDS, June 27, 2001, http://www.un.org/ga/aids/statements/docs/holyseeE.html.

2. Cited in Jill Haak Adels, *The Wisdom of the Saints: An Anthology* (New York: Oxford University Press, 1987), 57.

3. John Paul II, *Urbi et orbi* (December 25, 1988), n. 8.

4. Ethiopian Catholic Bishops, "Love As Our Main Tool of Overcoming HIV/AIDS," pastoral letter, Addis Ababa, February 25, 2007, 22.

5. Jean Pierre de Caussade, *Abandonment to Divine Providence*, ed. E. J. Strickland (New York: Cosimo, 2007), 94.

6. Thomas Merton, personal journal, March 19, 1958, cited in *A Year with Thomas Merton: Daily Meditations from His Journals*, ed. Jonathon Montaldo (New York: Harper Collins, 2004), 19.

7. Ethiopian Catholic Bishops, "Love as Our Main Tool," 23.

8. John Paul II, *Evangelium vitae* (March 25, 1995), n. 96, emphasis added.

9. Benedict XVI, interview with German broadcasters in preparation for his trip to Bavaria, Apostolic Palace of Castel Gandolfo, August 5, 2006, http://www.vatican.va/holy_father/ benedict_xvi/speeches/2006/august/documents/hf_ben -xvi_spe_20060805_intervista_en.html.

10. Anthony Fisher, "From *Evangelii Nuntiandi* to *Ecclesia in Oceania* and Beyond: After Twenty-Five Years of 'Evangelising the Culture' Where To from Here?" presented at the conference of the Fellowship of Catholic Scholars and the John Paul II Institute for Marriage and the Family, Melbourne, November 24, 2001.

11. Benedict XVI, homily, Munich, September 10, 2006.

12. Matthew Hanley, "Hope, Change, and AIDS," *Mercatornet*, December 1, 2009, http://www.mercatornet.com/articles/ view/hope_change_and_aids/.

13. John Paul II, *Veritatis splendor* (August 6, 1993), n. 106, original emphasis.

ACKNOWLEDGMENTS

We are grateful to so many people who have inspired us along the way—people who have dedicated their lives to caring for the sick and the orphans, to educating the young, and to engaging the wider culture.

We would like to thank Sister Dr. Miriam Duggan, F.M.S.A., one of the pioneers and architects of Uganda's successful response to the epidemic, and Dr. George Mulcaire-Jones, who generously reviewed the text and offered us valuable suggestions. Dr. Cristina Lopez, Barbara Larabell de Irala, Silvia Carlos Chilleron, and Asuncion Ruiz Ruiz also contributed generously, particularly early in this process, with references, citations, and editorial suggestions, among other things.

We are particularly grateful to The National Catholic Bioethics Center and its staff for their support in publishing this volume. Dr. Edward Furton, Rebecca Robinson, and Melanie Anderson each provided us with valuable suggestions and contributions throughout the process and were a pleasure to work with. David Mills provided an external editorial review which also sharpened our manuscript.

We would also like to thank our colleagues in the research and scientific community for their openness and collaboration, and for the efforts they have made in their pursuit of truth, even if it has sometimes cost them professionally.

We extend special and profound thanks to our families for their love and untiring support over the years.

MATTHEW HANLEY
JOKIN DE IRALA

BIBLIOGRAPHY

Abraham, Curtis. "UNAIDS and Myth of Condoms' Efficacy against AIDS." *East African*, February 7, 2009. http://www.theeastafrican.co .ke/news/-/2558/525956/-/rku48lz/-/index.html.

Ahmed, S., T. Lutalo, M. Wawer et al. "HIV Incidence and Sexually Transmitted Disease Prevalence Associated with Condom Use: A Population Study in Rakai, Uganda." *AIDS* 15.16 (November 9, 2009): 2171–2179.

Allen, John L. "The World from Rome." *National Catholic Reporter*, October 31, 2003. http://www.nationalcatholicreporter.org/word/ word103103.htm.

Allen, Tim, and Suzette Heald. "HIV/AIDS Policy in Africa: What Has Worked in Uganda and What Has Failed in Botswana?" *Journal of International Development* 16.8 (November 8, 2004): 1141–1154.

Alonso, Alvaro, and Jokin de Irala. "Strategies in HIV Prevention: The A-B-C Approach." *Lancet* 364.9431 (July 24–30, 2004): 1033.

Annan, Koffi A. *Message on the Occasion of World AIDS Day*. December 1, 2006. http://data.unaids.org/pub/PressStatement/2006/SG -worldaidsday2006.rev.pdf.

Autier, Philippe, Jean-Francois Doré, M.S. Cattaruzza et al. "Sunscreen Use, Wearing Clothes, and Number of Nevi in 6- to 7-Year-Old European Children. European Organization for Research and Treatment of Cancer Melanoma Cooperative Group." *Journal of the National Cancer Institute* 90.24 (December 16, 1998): 1873–1880.

Auvert, Bertran, Dirk Taljaard, Emmanuel Lagarde, Joëlle Sobngwi-Tambekou, Rémi Sitta, and Adrian Puren. "Randomized, Controlled Intervention Trial of Male Circumcision for Reduction of HIV Infection Risk: The ANRS 1265 Trial." *PLoS Medicine* 2.11 (November 2005): 1112–1122.

Bailey, Robert C., Stephen Moses, Coretet B. Parker et al. "Male Circumcision for HIV Prevention in Young Men in Kisumu, Kenya: A Randomized Controlled Trial." *Lancet* 369.9562 (February 24, 2007): 643–656.

Bello, G.A., J. Chipeta, and J. Aberle-Grasse. "Assessment of Trends in Biological and Behavioural Surveillance Data: Is There Any Evidence of Declining HIV Prevalence or Incidence in Malawi?" *Sexually Transmitted Infections* 82, suppl. 1 (April 2006): i9–i13.

Benedict XVI, Pope. Conclusion of the Meeting with the Bishops of Switzerland, November 9, 2006.

———. *Deus caritas est* (December 25, 2006).

———. Homily, Munich, September 10, 2006.

———. Interview with Broadcasters in Preparation for His Trip to Bavaria, Apostolic Palace of Castel Gandolfo, August 5, 2006.

———. *Truth and Tolerance: Christian Belief and World Religions.* San Francisco: Ignatius, 2004.

Bessinger, Ruth, Priscilla Akwara, and Daniel Halperin. *Sexual Behavior, HIV and Fertility Trends: A Comparative Analysis of Six Countries—Phase I of the ABC Study.* Washington, D.C.: USAID and MEASURE Evaluation, 2003.

Bosch, F. Xavier, Silvia de Sanjosé, Xavier Castellsagué et al. "Epidemiology of Human Papillomavirus Infections and Associations with Cervical Cancer: New Opportunities for Prevention." In *Papillomavirus Research: From Natural History to Vaccines and Beyond*, edited by M. Saveria Campo, 19–39. Wymondham, U.K.: Caister Academic, 2006.

Browder, Sue Ellin. "Why Condoms Will Never Stop AIDS in Africa." *Inside Catholic*, May 31, 2006. http://insidecatholic.com/Joomla/index.php?option=com_content&task=view&id=182&Itemid=12.

Bujo, Bénézet. "What Morality for the Problem of AIDS in Africa?" In *AIDS and the Church in Africa: To Shepherd the Church, Family of God in Africa in the Age of AIDS*, edited by Michael Czerny for the African Jesuit AIDS Network, 55–67. Nairobi: Pauline Publications, 2005.

Cassell, Michael M., Daniel T. Halperin, James D. Shelton, and David Stanton. "Risk Compensation: The Achilles' Heel of Innovations in HIV Prevention?" *British Medical Journal* 332.7541 (March 11, 2006): 605–607.

Centers for Disease Control and Prevention. "Achievements in Public Health: Reduction in Perinatal Transmission of HIV Infection—United States, 1985–2005." *Morbidity and Mortality Weekly Report* 55.21 (June 2, 2006): 592–597.

———. *HIV and Its Transmission*. Fact sheet, July 1999. http://www.cdc.gov/hiv/resources/factsheets/PDF/transmission.pdf.

*The Change Is On: Tools for Pure Living—Education for Life from Uganda to South Afric*a. DVD. Directed by Norman Servais. Metanoia Media, South Africa. 2008.

Cheluget, B., G. Baltazar, P. Orege, M. Ibrahim, L.H., Marum, and J. Stover. "Evidence for Population Level Declines in Adult HIV Prevalence in Kenya." *Sexually Transmitted Infection*s 82, suppl. 1 (April 2006): i21–i26.

Chesterton, C. K. "The Mercy of Mr. Arnold Bennett." In *Fancies versus Fads*. New York: Dodd, Mead, 1923. Reprint, Pomona Press, 2006.

Corbett, Elizabeth L., Beauty Makmure, Yin Bun Bheung et al. "HIV Incidence during a Cluster-Randomized Trial of Two Strategies Providing Voluntary Counselling and Testing at the Workplace, Zimbabwe." *AIDS* 21.4 (February 19, 2007): 483–489.

Corey, Lawrence. "Synergistic Copathogens: HIV-1 and HSV-2." *New England Journal of Medicine* 356.8 (February 22, 2007): 854–856.

Crawford, David. "Conjugal Love, Condoms, and HIV/AIDS." *Communio* 33.3 (Fall 2006): 505–512.

Czerny, Michael. "AIDS: Africa's Greatest Threat since the Slave Trade." *La Civiltà Cattolica* 3741 (May 6, 2006), http://www.jesuitaids.net/pdf/2006_Czerny_AIDS_Civilta_ENG_pdf.

———, ed., for the African Jesuit AIDS Network. *AIDS and the Church in Africa: To Shepherd the Church, Family of God in Africa in the Age of AIDS*. Nairobi: Pauline Publications, 2005.

————. "The Pope and AIDS in Africa: A Human and Spiritual Wake Up Call." *Thinking Faith*, March 25, 2009. http://www.thinkingfaith.org/articles/20090325_1.htm.

Dalrymple, Theodore. *Romancing Opiates*. New York: Encounter Books, 2006.

de Irala, Jokin. "Sexual Abstinence Education: What Is the Evidence We Need?" *British Medical Journal*. August 20, 2007. http://www.bmj.com/cgi/eletters/335/7613/248.

de Irala, Jokin, and Alvaro Alonso. "Changes in Sexual Behaviors to Prevent HIV: The Need for Comprehensive Information." *Lancet* 368.9549 (November 18, 2006): 1749–1750.

Dickson, Nigel, Charlotte Paul, Peter Herbison, and Phil Silva. "First Sexual Intercourse: Age, Coercion, and Later Regrets Reported by a Birth Cohort." *British Medical Journal* 316.7124 (January 3, 1998): 29–33.

DiClemente, Ralph J., Richard A. Crosby, Gina M. Wingwood, Delia L. Lang, Larua F. Salazar, and Sherry D. Broadwell. "Reducing Risk Exposures to Zero and Not Having Multiple Partners: Findings That Inform Evidence-Based Practices Designed to Prevent STD Acquisition." *International Journal of STD and AIDS* 16.12 (December 2005): 816–818.

Downing, Raymond. "African Perspective on AIDS Crisis Differs from West." *National Catholic Reporter*, January 21, 2005.

Duggan, Miriam. "Combating the Spread of AIDS." In *Culture of Life—Culture of Death*, edited by Luke Gormally, 257–267. London: Linacre Center, 2002.

Dulles, Avery Cardinal. "Can Philosophy Be Christian?" *First Things* 102 (April 2000): 24–29.

Eberstadt, Mary. "The Vindication of *Humanae vitae*." *First Things* 185 (August–September 2008).

Epstein, Helen. "Africa's Lethal Web Net of AIDS: The Quiet Acceptance of Informal Polygamy Is Spreading the Risk." *Los Angeles Times*, April 15, 2007. http://articles.latimes.com/2007/apr/15/opinoin/op-epstein15.

Ethiopian Catholic Bishops. *Love as Our Main Tool of Overcoming HIV/AIDS*. Pastoral letter, Addis Ababa, February 25, 2007.

FASU Consultancy and Maternal Life International. *AIDS Cultural Change Programme 2001–2006: Operation Phase 2004–2006.* Lilongwe, Malawi, and Butte, MT: FAMLI, 2006.

Fauci, Anthony S. "A Policy Cocktail for Fighting HIV." *Washington Post*, April 16, 2009.

Finnis, John. *Fundamentals of Ethics.* Oxford, U.K.: Clarendon, 1984.

Fisher, Anthony. "The Catholic Church and the Drug Crisis." Talk given to the Endeavour Forum at St Joseph's Hall, Malvern, Victoria, Australia, February 10, 2000.

———. "Cooperation, Condoms and HIV." Henkels Lecture at the Institute of Bioethics at Franciscan University of Steubenville, Ohio, September 10, 2008.

———. "From Evangelii Nuntiandi to Ecclesia in Oceania and Beyond: After Twenty-Five Years of 'Evangelising the Culture' Where To from Here?" Paper presented at the conference of the Fellowship of Catholic Scholars and the John Paul II Institute for Marriage and the Family, Melbourne, November 24, 2001.

———. "Moral Theology from Vatican II to John Paul II." Lecture to the Australian Confraternity of Catholic Clergy National Conference, Galong, New South Wales, Australia, July 14, 1998.

———. "The Pastoral Application on the Theology of the Body." Centrecare Natural Family Planning Conference, Randwick, Australia, October 23, 2004. http://www.sydney.catholic.org.au/people/bishop_anthony_fisher/addresses/2004/20041023_819.shtml.

———. Speech at the Graduation Mass, University of Notre Dame, Fremantle, Australia, July 16, 2006.

———. "Theology of the Body: Love, Life, Sex—The Good News about Sexuality." Paper presented at the seminar of the Australian Council of Natural Family Planning, Sydney, October 10, 2003.

Garrett, Laurie. "The Lessons of HIV/AIDS." *Foreign Affairs* 84.4 (July–August 2005): 51–64.

Genuis, Stephen J., and Shelagh K. Genuis. "Managing the Sexually Transmitted Disease Pandemic: A Time for Reevaluation." *American Journal of Obstetrics and Gynecology* 191.4 (October 2004): 1103–1112.

George, Robert. "A Clash of Orthodoxies." *First Things* 95 (August–September 1999): 33–40.

———. "Sweet Reason." Review. *First Things* 159 (January 2006): 56–59.

Glick, Peter. *Reproductive Health and Behavior, HIV/AIDS, and Poverty in Africa.* SAGA Working Paper. Ithaca, NY: Strategies and Analysis for Growth and Access, May 2007. http://www.saga.cornell.edu/images/wp219.pdf.

———. *Scaling up HIV Voluntary Counseling and Testing in Africa: What Can Evaluation Studies Tell Us about Potential Prevention Impacts?* SAGA Working Paper. Ithaca, NY: Strategies and Analysis for Growth and Access, March 2005. http://pdf.dec.org/pdf_docs/PNADC113.pdf.

Gray, Ronald H., Godfrey Kigozi, David Serwadda et al. "Male Circumcision for HIV Prevention in Men in Rakai, Uganda: A Randomised Trial." *Lancet* 369.9562 (February 24, 2007): 657–666.

Green, Edward C. "ABC: Expanding Prevention Models to Generalized Epidemics." Presentation. May 25, 2005. http://coburn.senate.gov/oversight/?FuseAction=Files.View&FileStore_id=dd4e2cc9-89d7-4db9-99fa-1756942bf539.

———. "AIDS in Africa—A Betrayal: The One Success Story Is Now Threatened by U.S. Aid Bureaucrats." *Weekly Standard* 10.19 (January 31, 2005). http://www.weeklystandard.com/Content/Protected/Articles/000/000/005/172wwqzc.asp?pg=1.

———. "Culture Clash and AIDS Prevention." *Responsive Community* 13.4 (2003): 4–9.

———. *Faith-Based Organizations: Contributions to HIV Prevention.* Washington, D.C.: USAID/Washington and Synergy Project, September 2003.

———. Interview with *Ilsussidiario*, March 23, 2009. http://www.ilsussidiario.net/articolo.aspx?articolo=14614.

———. "The Pope May Be Right." *Washington Post*, March 29, 2009. http://www.washingtonpost.com/wp-dyn/content/article/2009/03/27/AR2009032702825_pf.html.

———. "Poverty Does Not Mean That Effective AIDS Prevention Is Impossible." *Share the World's Resources*, January 29, 2006.

http://www.stwr.org/health-education-shelter/poverty-does-not
-mean-that-effective-aids-prevention-is-impossible.html.

——— . *Rethinking AIDS Prevention: Learning from Successes in Developing Countries*. Westport, CT: Praeger, 2003.

——— "A Summary of ABC Evidence." Presentation to the Presidential Advisory Council on HIV/AIDS, March 29, 2004. http://www.ccih.org/resources/ABCplus/research/abc/ABC-expanding-prevention-models.pdf.

——— . Testimony before the U.S. Senate Subcommittee on Africa. May 19, 2003.

Green, Edward C., Daniel T. Halperin, Vinand Nantulya, and Janice A. Hogle. "Uganda's HIV Prevention Success: The Role of Sexual Behavior Change and the National Response," *AIDS Behavior* 10.4 (July 2006): 335–346.

Green, Edward C., and Allison Herling. *The ABC Approach to Preventing the Sexual Transmission of AIDS: Common Questions and Answers*. McLean, VA: Christian Connections for International Health and Medical Service Corporation International, February 2007. http://www.harvardaidsprp.org/research/Green&Herling_ABC_Approach_Feb07(2).pdf.

Gregson, Simon, Geoffrey P. Garnett, Constance A. Nyamukapa et al. "HIV Decline Associated with Behavior Change in Eastern Zimbabwe." *Science* 311.5761 (February 3, 2006): 664–666.

Grisez, Germain. *The Way of the Lord Jesus*, vol. 3, *Difficult Moral Questions*. Quincy, IL: Franciscan Press, 1997.

Hallett, Timothy B., J. Aberle-Grasse, G. Bellot et al. "Declines in HIV Prevalence Can Be Associated with Changing Sexual Behaviour in Uganda, Urban Kenya, Zimbabwe, and Urban Haiti." *Sexually Transmitted Infections* 82, suppl. 1 (April 2006): i1–i8.

Halperin, Daniel. "Why Is HIV Prevalence So High in Southern Africa, and What Can Be Done about It?" Presentation at Harvard Medical School, Boston, June 17, 2008.

Halperin, Daniel T., M. Steiner, M. Cassell et al. "The Time Has Come for Common Ground on Preventing Sexual Transmission of HIV." *Lancet* 364.9449 (November 27–December 3, 2004): 1913–1915.

Hanley, Matthew. "AIDS and 'Technical Solutions': First Change Sexual Behavior." *Ethics & Medics* 33.12 (December 2008): 1–3.

———. "Hope, Change, and AIDS." *MercatorNet*, December 1, 2009. http://www.mercatornet.com/articles/view/hope_change _and_aids/.

———. "A Realistic Strategy for Fighting African AIDS." *MercatorNet*, February 28, 2008. http://www.mercatornet.com/articles/a_realistic _strategy_for_fighting_african_aids.

Hearst, Norman, and Sanny Chen. "Condom Promotion for AIDS Prevention in the Developing World: Is It Working?" *Studies in Family Planning* 35.1 (March 2004): 39–47.

Helleringer, Stéphane, and Hans-Peter Kohler. "Sexual Network Struc-ture and the Spread of HIV in Africa: Evidence from Likoma Island, Malawi." *AIDS* 21.17 (November 12, 2007): 2323–2332.

Hogle, Janice A., ed., *What Happened in Uganda? Declining HIV Prevalence, Behavior Change and the National Response*. Washington, D.C.: U.S. Agency for International Development, September 2002. http://www.usaid.gov/pop_health/aids/Countries/africa/ uganda_report.pdf.

Holbrook, Richard. "Sorry, But AIDS Testing Is Critical." *Washington Post*, January 4, 2006.

International Labour Organization. *Malawi National HIV/ AIDS Policy*. June 2003. http://www.ilo.org/public/english/ protection/trav/aids/laws/malawi1.pdf.

John, Minnie, Marla J. Keller, Ehsan H. Fam et al. "Cervicovaginal Secre-tions Contribute to Innate Resistance to Herpes Simplex Virus Infec-tion." *Journal of Infectious Disease* 192.10 (2005): 1731–1740.

John Paul II, Pope. Address to the Diplomatic Community in Nairobi (May 7, 1980).

———. *Evangelium vitae* (March 25, 1995).

———. *Familiaris consortio* (November 22, 1981).

———. *Fides et ratio* (September 14, 1998).

———. *Letter to Families* (February 2, 1994).

———. *Redemptor Hominis* (March 4, 1979).

———. *Urbi et orbi* (December 25, 1988).

———. *Veritatis splendor* (August 6, 1993).

Joint U.N. Program on HIV/AIDS. *2006 Report on the Global AIDS Epidemic*. Geneva, May 2006. http://data.unaids.org/pub/Global Report/2006/2006_GR_CH02_en.pdf.

―――. *2008 Report on the Global AIDS Epidemic*. Geneva, August 2008. http://data.unaids.org/pub/GlobalReport/2008/jc1510 _2008_global_report_pp29_62_en.pdf.

Joint U.N. Program on HIV/AIDS and World Health Organization. *AIDS Epidemic Update: December 2003* (UNAIDS/03.39E). http://data.unaids.org/Publications/IRC-pub06/JC943-Epi Update2003_en.pdf.

―――. *AIDS Epidemic Update: December 2005* (UNAIDS/05.19E). http://www.unaids.org/epi/2005/doc/EPIupdate2005_pdf_en/ epi-update2005_en.pdf.

―――. *AIDS Epidemic Update: December 2007* (UNAIDS/07.27E). http://data.unaids.org/pub/EPISlides/2007/2007_epiupdate _en.pdf.

Kajubi, Phoebe, Moses R. Kamya, Sarah Kamya, Sanny Chen, Willi McFarland, and Norman Hearst. "Increasing Condom Use without Reducing HIV Risk: Results of a Controlled Community Trial in Uganda." *Journal of Acquired Immune Deficiency Syndromes* 40.1 (September 1, 2005): 77–82.

Kayirangwa, E., J. Hanson, L. Munyakazi, and A. Kabeja. "Current Trends in Rwanda's HIV/AIDS Epidemic." *Sexually Transmitted Infections* 82, suppl. 1 (April 2006): i27–i31.

Kelly, Michael. "The Church as Servant, Teacher and Prophet in Today's HIV/AIDS Crisis." *Jesuit Centre for Theological Reflection* 44 (Second Quarter 2000), http://www.jesuitaids.net/go.aspx?B1=htm/ Church%20as%20Leader.htm&RZ=1&TL=1.

Kenya Catholic Church HIV and AIDS Taskforce. *This We Teach and Do*. Nairobi: Kenya Episcopal Conference—Catholic Secretariat, 2006.

Kirkkola, Anna-Leena, Kari Mattila, and Irma Virjo. "Problems with Condoms: A Population-Based Study among Finnish Men and Women." *European Journal of Contraception and Reproductive Health Care* 10.2 (June 2005): 87–92.

Kristof, Nicholas D. "The Pope and AIDS." *New York Times*, May 8, 2005.

Kurisanani Team, Diocese of Tzaneen, *HIV/AIDS Response—2006 Report on Activities*. Limpopo, South Africa, 2006.

Lawler, Kay. *Education for Life: A Behaviour Process*. Masaka, Uganda: Kitovu Hospital, 1997.

L'Engle, Kelly, Jane Brown, and Kristin Kenneavy. "The Mass Media Are an Important Context for Adolscents' Sexual Behavior." *Journal of Adolescent Health* 38.3 (2006): 186–192.

Leclerc-Madlala, Suzanne. "Prevention Means More Than Condoms." *Mail and Guardian*, October 4, 2002. http://www.aegis.com/news/dmg/2002/MG021003.html.

———. "The Beliefs and Behaviors That Are Driving AIDS Have to Change." *Sunday Independent* [South Africa], March 12, 2006. http://www.sundayindependent.co.za/index.php.

Legardy, Jennifer K., Maurizio Macaluso, Lynn Artz, and Ilene Brill. "Do Participant Characteristics Influence the Effectiveness of Behavioral Interventions? Promoting Condom Use to Women." *Sexually Transmitted Diseases* 32.11 (November 2005): 665–671.

Liebowitz, Jeremy. *The Impact of Faith-Based Organizations on HIV/AIDS Prevention and Mitigation in Africa*. Prepared for the Health Economics and HIV/AIDS Research Division, University of Natal, Durban, South Africa, October 2002. http://www.heard.org.za/heard-resources/assortment.

Lopez, Alan D., Colin D. Mathers, Majid Ezzati et al. "Global and Regional Burden of Disease and Risk Factors, 2001: Systematic Analysis of Population Health Data." *Lancet* 367.9524 (May 27, 2006): 1747–1757.

Low-Beer, Daniel. "Global Failures and Local Successes in HIV Prevention." Online letter to the editor. *British Medical Journal*, July 9, 2003. http://www.bmj.com/cgi/eletters/326/7403/1389#34209.

———. "Going Face to Face with AIDS: This Is a Routinely Avoidable Disease." *Financial Times*, November 28, 2003.

Low-Beer, Daniel, and Rand L. Stoneburner. "Behavior and Communication Change in Reducing HIV: Is Uganda Unique?" *African Journal of AIDS Research* 2.1 (May 2003): 9–21.

Lozano-Barragán, Javier Lozano. Statement on HIV/AIDS to the U.N. General Assembly, Twenty-sixth Special Session, June 27, 2001. http://www.un.org/ga/aids/statements/docs/holyseeE.html.

Bibliography

MacIntyre, Alasdair. *After Virtue: A Study in Moral Theory*. Notre Dame: IN: University of Notre Dame Press, 1981.

Mahomva, A., S. Greby, S. Dube et al. "HIV Prevalence and Trends from Data in Zimbabwe: 1997–2004." *Sexually Transmitted Infections* 82, suppl. 1 (April 2006): i42–i47.

Mahy, Mary, and Neeru Gupta. "Trends and Differentials in Adolescent Reproductive Behavior in Sub-Saharan Africa." In *DHS Analytical Studies 3*, Macro International and Measure DHS Project. Calverton, MD: ORC Macro, 2002.

Martinez-Gonzalez, M.A., and Jokin de Irala. "Preventive Medicine and the Catastrophic Failures of Public Health: We Fail Because We Are Late" [in Spanish]. *Medicina Clínica* 124.17 (May 7, 2005): 656–660.

Masanjala, Winford. "The Poverty-HIV/AIDS Nexus in Africa: A Livelihood Approach." *Social Science and Medicine* 64.5 (March 2007): 1032–1041.

Maternal Life International with Catholic Relief Services. *The Faithful House: Building Strong Families to Affirm Life and Avoid Risk*. DVD. 2005.

Matovu, Joseph K. B., Ronald H. Gray, Noah Kiwanuka, et al. "Repeat Voluntary HIV Counseling and Testing (VCT), Sexual Risk Behavior and HIV Incidence in Rakai, Uganda." *AIDS and Behavior* 11.1 (January 2007): 71–78.

Meeking, Basil. "Proclaim the Truth through Love: A Comment on Deus caritas est." *Logos* 10.3 (Summer 2007): 91–104.

Mekonnen, Yared, Eduard Sanders, Mathias Aklilu, et al. "Evidence of Changes in Sexual Behavior among Male Factory Workers in Ethiopia." *AIDS* 17.2 (2003): 223–231.

Mishra, Vinod, Rathavuth Hong, Simona Bignami-Van Assche, and Bernard Barrere. *The Role of Partner Reduction and Faithfulness in HIV Prevention in Sub-Saharan Africa: Evidence from Cameroon, Rwanda, Uganda, and Zimbabwe*. DHS working paper 61, Macro International for USAID. January 2009. http://www.measuredhs.com/pubs/pdf/WP61/WP61.pdf.

Mishra, Vinod, Simona Bignami, Robert Greener, et al. *A Study of the Association of HIV Infection with Wealth in Sub-Saharan Africa*. DHS working paper 31, Macro International for USAID. January 2007. http://www.measuredhs.com/pubs/pdf/WP31/WP31.

Mishra, Vinod, Simona Bignami-Van Assche, Robert Greener et al. "HIV Infection Does Not Disproportionately Affect the Poorer in Sub-Saharan Africa." *AIDS* 21, suppl. 7 (November 2007): s17–s28.

Munro, Alison. "Responsibility: The Prevention of HIV/AIDS." In *Responsibility in a Time of AIDS: A Pastoral Response by Catholic Theologians and AIDS Activists in Southern Africa*, edited by Stuart C. Bate, 2–18. Pietermaritzburg, South Africa: Cluster Publications, 2003.

Museveni, Yoweri Kaguta. "AIDS and Its Impact on the Health and Social Service and Infrastructure in Developing Countries." Speech by the President of Uganda at the International Conference on AIDS, Florence, Italy, June 16, 1991.

Napier, Wilfrid Cardinal, ed. *Youth Alive: A Workbook for the Youth in the Southern African Catholic Bishops' Conference*. Pretoria, South Africa: SACBC, 2007.

Neill, Rosemary. "A Catholic Culture of Death." *Australian*, May 7, 2005.

Oxman, Andrew D., John N. Lavis, and Atle Fretheim. "Use of Evidence in WHO Recommendations." *World Hospitals and Health Services* 43.2 (2007):14–20, reprinted from *Lancet* 369.9576 (June 2, 2007): 1883–1889.

Pacholczyk, Tadeusz. "Conundrum with Condoms." *Making Sense Out of Bioethics* column, June 2006, National Catholic Bioethics Center, http://www.ncbcenter.org/NetCommunity/Page.aspx?pid=284.

Parker, Joan, Ira Singh, and Kelly Hattel. *The Role of Microfinance in the Fight against HIV/AIDS: A Report to UNAIDS*. Bethesda, MD: Development Alternatives, September 15, 2000. http://www.microfinance gateway.org/gm/document-1.9.29154/2737_file_02737.pdf.

Paul VI, Pope. *Humanae vitae* (July 25, 1968).

Paz-Bailey, Gabriela, Emilia H. Koumans, Maya Sternberg et al. "The Effect of Correct and Consistent Condom Use on Chlamydial and Gonococcal Infection among Urban Adolescents." *Archives of Pediatrics and Adolescent Medicine* 159.6 (2005): 536–542.

Pell, George Cardinal. "Varieties of Intolerance: Religious and Secular." Inaugural Hilary Term Lecture, Oxford University Newman Society, March 6, 2009. http://users.ox.ac.uk/~newman/varieties ofintolerance.pdf.

Bibliography

Piot, Peter. "AIDS: The Need for an Exceptional Response to an Unprecedented Crisis." A Presidential Fellows lecture, November 20, 2003. http://data.unaids.org/Media/Speeches 02/Piot_WorldBank_20Nov03_en.pdf.

———. "Global Health: America's Response." Interview by David Brancaccio. *NOW* documentary transcript, PBS (November 4, 2005). http://www.pbs.org/now/transcript/transcriptNOW GL_full.html.

———. Keynote address to the Twenty-eighth Session Symposium, *Nutrition and HIV/AIDS*, Nairobi, Kenya, April 3–4, 2001. U.N. Administrative Committee on Coordination, Sub-Committee on Nutrition. Nutrition Policy Paper 20. Geneva: UN ACC/SCN, 2001.

"The Pope on Condoms and AIDS." Editorial. *New York Times*, March 17, 2009.

Population, Health and Nutrition Information (PHNI) Project. *The ABCs of HIV Prevention: Report of a USAID Technical Meeting on Behavior Change Approaches to Primary Prevention of HIV/AIDS*. Washington, D.C.: USAID, September 17, 2002. http://www .usaid.gov/our_work/global_health/aids/TechAreas/prevention/ abc.pdf.

Potts, Malcolm, Daniel T. Halperin, Douglas Kirby et al. "Reassessing HIV Prevention." *Science* 320.5877 (May 9, 2008): 749–750.

Potts, Malcolm, and Julia Walsh. "Tackling India's HIV Epidemic: Lessons from Africa." *British Medical Journal* 326.7403 (June 21, 2003): 1389–1392.

Revzina, N. V., and R. J. DiClemente, "Prevalence and Incidence of Human Papillomavirus Infection in Women in the USA: A Systematic Review." *International Journal of STD and AIDS* 16.8 (2005): 528–537.

Richens, John, John Imrie, and Andrew Copas. "Condoms and Seat Belts: The Parallels and the Lessons." *Lancet* 355.9201 (January 29, 2000): 400–403.

Richens, John, John Imrie, and Helen Weiss. "Human Immuno-deficiency Virus Risk: Is It Possible to Dissuade People from Having Unsafe Sex?" *Journal of the Royal Statistical Society: Series A* 166.2 (June 2003): 207–215.

Russell, Ben. "It's Time You Faced Up to AIDS, Tony Blair Tells Church Leaders." *Independent* [Ireland], December 2, 2006. http://www .independent.ie/national-news/its-time-you-faced-up-to-aids-tony -blair-tells-church-leaders-6265.html.

Ruteikara, Sam. "Let My People Go, AIDS Profiteers." *Washington Post*, June 30, 2008.

Sangani Prerana, George Rutherford, and Gail E. Kennedy. "Population-Based Interventions for Reducing Sexually Transmitted Infections, Including HIV Infection." *Cochrane Database of Systematic Reviews*, issue 3, article CD001220, 2004.

Santamaria, Joseph Natalin. "Drug Abuse: The Battle over Harm Minimisation." H.R. Francis Memorial Lecture, May 2003, revised November 26, 2004. Drug Advisory Council of Australia. http://www.daca.org.au/rehab/BA_santamaria.htm.

Shelton, James D. "Confessions of a Condom Lover." *Lancet* 368.9551 (December 2, 2006): 1947–1949.

———. "Ten Myths and One Truth about Generalized HIV Epidemics." *Lancet* 370.9602 (December 1, 2007): 1809–1811.

Shelton, James D., Michael M. Cassell, and Jacob Adetunji. "Is Poverty or Wealth at the Root of HIV?" *Lancet* 366.9491 (September 24–30, 2005): 1057–1058.

Sheth, Shirish S. "Missing Female Births in India." *Lancet* 367.9506 (January 21, 2006): 185–186.

Shisana, Olive, Thomas Rehle, Leickness Simbayi, et al. *South African National HIV Prevalence, HIV Incidence, Behaviour and Communication Survey, 2005*. Cape Town, South Africa: Human Sciences Research Council, 2005. http://www.hsrcpress.ac.za/product.php ?productid=2134.

Širinskienė, Agnė. "Manifestation of Different Ethical Theories in the Content of HIV Prevention" [in Polish]. *Journal of Religious Science* 21.49 (2007): 153–162.

Smith, Janet. "Chastity." In *Our Sunday Visitor's Encyclopedia of Catholic Doctrine*, edited by Russell Shaw, 92. Huntington, IN: OSV, 1997.

Southern African Development Community. *Expert Think Tank Meeting on HIV Prevention in High-Prevalence Countries in Southern Africa: Report, Maseru, Lesotho, May 10–12, 2006*. Gaborone,

Botswana: SADC, July 2006. http://data.unaids.org/pub/Report/2006/20060601_sadc_meeting_report_en.pdf.

Sowing in Tears. Documentary on the comprehensive response of the Diocese of Tzaneen, Limpopo Province, to the HIV/AIDS pandemic. DVD. Directed by Norman Servais. Metanoia Media, South Africa. 2007.

Stammers, T. "As Easy as ABC? Primary Prevention of Sexually Transmitted Infections." *Postgraduate Medicine Journal* 81.955 (May 2005): 273—275.

Stanton, David. "Evidence vs. Conventional Wisdom: AIDS Prevention in the Twenty-first Century." Presentation at the Johns Hopkins University, Baltimore, Maryland, March 13, 2009.

Stolte, Ineke G. John B.F. de Wit, Marion Kolader et al. "Association between 'Safer Sex Fatigue' and Rectal Gonorrhea Is Mediated by Unsafe Sex with Casual Partners among HIV-Positive Homosexual Men." *Sexually Transmitted Diseases* 33.4 (April 2006): 201–208.

Stoneburner, Rand, and Daniel Low-Beer. "Population-Level HIV Declines and Behavioral Risk Avoidance in Uganda." *Science* 304.5671 (April 30, 2004): 714–718.

Sylva, Douglas A. "AIDS and the Ideological Barrier: The Threat to Sexual Liberation." *Ethics & Medics* 33.12 (December 2008).

Tan, Andy, Thato Letsatsi, Joshua Volle, and Jim Foreit for USAID. *A Baseline Survey of Multiple and Concurrent Sexual Partnerships among Basotho Men in Lesotho*. C-Change/Academy for Educational Development, July 2009.

Tanzania Commission for AIDS (TACAIDS), National Bureau of Statistics (NBS), and ORC Macro. *Tanzania HIV/AIDS Indicator Survey 2003–04*. Calverton, MD: TACAIDS, NBS, and ORC, 2005.

Taylor, Charles. *A Secular Age*. Cambridge, MA: Belknap Press of Harvard University Press, 2007.

Thickstun, Patricia, and Kate Hendricks, eds. *Evidence That Demands Action: Comparing Risk Avoidance and Risk Reduction Strategies for HIV Prevention*, with papers by Edward C. Green, Rand L. Stoneburner and Daniel Low-Beer, and Norman Hearst and Sanny Chen. Austin, TX: Medical Institute for Sexual Health, 2004.

https://secure.digital-community.com/english/medinstitute.org/
includes/downloads/abc.pdf?PHPSESSID=63bb6283d34c3a32
51664333d31acd74.

Thurow, Roger. "AIDS Fuels Famine in Africa." *Wall Street Journal*,
July 9, 2003.

Tun, Waimar, David D. Celentano, David Vlahov, and Steffanie A.
Strathdee. "Attitudes toward HIV Treatments Influence Unsafe
Sexual and Injection Practices among Injecting Drug Users." *AIDS*
17.13 (September 5, 2003): 1953–1962.

United Nations Administrative Committee on Coordination, Sub-
Committee on Nutrition. *Nutrition and HIV/AIDS*. Report
of Twenty-eighth Session Symposium, Nairobi, Kenya, April
3–4, 2001. Nutrition Policy Paper 20. Geneva: UN ACC/SCN,
2001.

United Nations Development Program. Human Development Report
2005: International Cooperation at a Crossroads—Air, Trade and
Security in an Unequal World. New York: UNDP, 2005. http://
hdr.undp.org/en/media/HDR05_complete.pdf.

United Nations General Assembly, Twenty-sixth Special Session. *Declaration of Commitment on HIV/AIDS*. August 2, 2001 (A/RES/S-26/2).
http://www.un.org/ga/aids/docs/aress262.pdf.

United Nations Population Division. *HIV/AIDS Awareness and Behaviour*. (ST/ESA/SER.A/209), 2002.

United States Agency for International Development (USAID).
*The "ABCs" of HIV Prevention: Report of the USAID Technical
Meeting on Behavior Change Approaches to Primary Prevention of
HIV/AIDS*. Washington, D.C., September 17, 2002. http://www.
usaid.gov/our_work/global_health/aids/TechAreas/prevention/
abc.pdf.

United States Congress. Senate. Committee on Foreign Relations. *Fighting AIDS in Uganda: What Went Right? Hearing
before the Committee on Foreign Relations*. 108th Congress, 1st
session, May 19, 2003. http://foreign.senate.gov/hearings/2003/
hrg030519p.html.

Vaccarella, Salvatore, Silvia Franceschi, Rolando Herrero et al. "Sexual
Behavior, Condom Use, and Human Papillomavirus: Pooled
Analysis of the IARC Human Papillomavirus Prevalence Surveys."

Bibliography

Cancer Epidemiology, Biomarkers and Prevention 15.2 (February 2006): 326–333.

Vatican Council II. *Gaudium et spes* (December 7, 1965).

Von Hildebrand, Alice. "Why Truth and Charity Are Inseparable." *AD2000* 20.6 (July 2007).

Walker, Martin. "The Geopolitics of Sexual Frustration." *Foreign Policy* (March–April 2006).

Weigel, George. *Witness to Hope: The Biography of Pope John Paul II.* New York: Harper Collins, 1999.

Weinhardt, Lance S., Michael P. Cary, Blair T. Johnson, and Nicole L. Bickham. "Effects of HIV Counseling and Testing on Sexual Risk Behavior: A Meta-Analytic Review of Published Research, 1985–1997." *American Journal of Public Health* 89.9 (1999): 1397–1405.

Weller, Susan C., and Karen R. Davis. "Condom Effectiveness in Reducing Heterosexual HIV Transmission." *Cochrane Database of Systematic Reviews*, issue 3, article CD003255, 2001.

West, Christopher. *Theology of the Body Explained*. Boston: Pauline Books and Media, 2003.

Wilson, David, and Joy de Beyer. "Male Circumcision: Evidence and Implications." *World Bank HIV/AIDS Monitoring and Evaluation: Getting Results.* World Bank Global HIV/AIDS Program, March 2006.

Wilson, David, and Daniel T. Halperin. "'Know Your Epidemic, Know Your Response': A Useful Approach If We Get It Right." *Lancet* 372.9637 (August 9, 2008): 423–426.

Wilson, David. "Partner Reduction and the Prevention of HIV/AIDS." *British Medical Journal* 328.7444 (April 10, 2004): 848–849.

Wilson Favors, Therese. "Three Popes Who Came from Africa." *Catholic Review*, April 28, 2005.

Winer, Rachel L., James P. Hughes, Qinghua Feng et al. "Condom Use and the Risk of Genital Human Papillomavirus Infection in Young Women." *New England Journal of Medicine* 354.25 (June 22, 2006): 2645–2654.

Women of Uganda Network. *The Arusha Commitments of Gender and HIV/AIDS: From Policy to Practice in East Africa.* Draft. 2003.

http://www.wougnet.org/Documents/UNIFEM/arusha_gen
derhiv.html.

World AIDS Campaign. *Stop AIDS—Keep the Promise: 2005
and Beyond*, 2005. http://data.unaids.org/WAC/wac05_over
view_en.pdf.

World Health Organization. *Global Prevalence and Incidence of
Selected Curable Sexually Transmitted Infections: Overview and
Estimates*. Geneva: WHO, 2001. http://www.who.int/hiv/pub/
sti/who_hiv_aids_2001.02.pdf.

———. *Priority Interventions: HIV/AIDS Prevention, Treatment and
Care in the Health Sector*, version 1.2. Geneva, 2009. http://www
.who.int/hiv/pub/priority_interventions_web.pdf.

Wojtyla, Karol. *Love and Responsibility*. San Francisco: Ignatius Press,
1993.

Wrong, Michela. "Blood of Innocents on His Hands." *New Statesman*, April 11, 2005.

AUTHORS

After earning his master's degree in public health from Emory University in Atlanta in 2000, MATTHEW HANLEY worked as an HIV/AIDS Technical Advisor for Catholic Relief Services until 2008. He specialized in HIV prevention and in home-based care for people living with HIV/AIDS, and has traveled extensively in Africa. He currently writes on matters of public health, ethics, and culture from California.

DR. JOKIN DE IRALA is deputy director of the Department of Preventive Medicine and Public Health and the Institute of Sciences for the Family at the University of Navarra in Pamplona, Spain. He holds a medical degree and a doctoral degree in medicine from the University of Navarra, a master's degree in public health from the University of Dundee (Scotland, 1987), and a second doctoral degree, in epidemiology, from the University of Massachusetts. He is an active teacher and has published numerous books and scientific papers.

Hanley and de Irala have been collaborating closely since 2005.

INDEX

Index